Vitality Plan

Vitality Plan

Deborah Bull

LONDON • NEW YORK • MOSCOW • SYDNEY

www.dk.com

A DORLING KINDERSLEY BOOK

www.dk.com

Project Editor Monica Chakraverty

Art Editor Robert Ford

Editor David Summers

Designer Claudia Norris

Senior Art Editor Tracey Clarke

DTP Designer Karen Ruane

Managing Editor Susannah Marriott/Mary Ling

Managing Art Editor Toni Kay

Photographers Dave King, Andy Crawford, Gary Ombler

Production Manager Maryann Rogers

"Nobody gets it wrong on purpose."
(after Socrates)

For Torje, who made sense of it all.

First published in Great Britain in 1998 by
Dorling Kindersley Limited,
9 Henrietta Street, London WC2E 8PS

First published as a Dorling Kindersley paperback in 1999

2 4 6 8 10 9 7 5 3

A CIP catalogue record for this book is available
from the British Library.

ISBN 0 7513 0570 7

Reproduced in Singapore by Colourscan
Printed and bound in Singapore by Star Standard Industries (Pte.) Ltd.

Contents

FOREWORD 6

INTRODUCTION 7

Weight Loss: The Facts 10

*Understanding how the body works and
how to work with it to lose weight*

The Myths 12

The Facts 14

Using Energy 16

Diet or Exercise? 18

What is Exercise? 19

What Type of Exercise? 20

Reading Your Heart Rate 22

Energy for Life 24

A complete nutrition guide explains the fundamentals of a healthy diet

The Low-down on Calories 26
Carbohydrates 28
Protein 30
Fat 32
Vitamins & Minerals 34
Water 36
Striking a Balance 38
How to Read Food Labels 40
Seven Point Plan 41

The Good Food Guides 42

The Good Breakfast Guide 43
The Good Lunch Guide 44
The Good Dinner Guide 46
The Good Snack Guide 48

Total Fitness Plan 50

A fitness package to last a lifetime, with an effective exercise routine to tone the whole body

Getting the Right Gear 52
When to Exercise 54
The Pre-exercise Plan 55

The Fitness Plan 56

Warm Up 57
Light Stretch 58
Aerobic Exercise 60
5-minute Cool Down 63

Strength Training 64

Abdominals 65 ▪ Back Extensions 66
Chair Dips 68 ▪ Hamstrings 70
Biceps 72 ▪ Arabesque 74
Inner Thigh 76 ▪ Deltoid 78

Stretches 80

Inner Thigh 81 ▪ Hip Flexor 82
Front Thigh 84 ▪ Hamstrings 85
Upper Calf 86 ▪ Lower Calf 87
Side Stretch 88 ▪ Cat Stretch 90
Hanging Stretch 91

GLOSSARY 92
INDEX 93 – 95
USEFUL ADDRESSES 96
ACKNOWLEDGMENTS 96

Foreword

WHENEVER I WATCH DEBORAH BULL DANCE, I am amazed by how terrific she looks and how much energy she seems to have. *The Vitality Plan* tells you just how she does it. In this book, she gives you the information you need to help you maximize your energy yet still control your weight.

In all the years I've been modelling, I've come across many weird and wonderful diets. Yet in the long run, none of them ever work because, as Deborah says, losing weight is not about the things you should not do, it's about the things you should do. You can stay slim without starving yourself, and you don't need expensive gyms or exercise equipment to keep fit. Like me, Deborah follows Torje Eike's Total Fitness Plan, a routine I have relied on for years to keep me in shape. If you are fed up of dieting but want to lose weight – for life – I can't think of two people better equipped to tell you how.

JERRY HALL

Fit for Life

ONE IN EVERY FOUR ADULTS in Western Europe is overweight; in the United States, this figure is as high as one in three. It is hardly surprising that we have an obsession with diet. For some of us, getting thin has become an all-consuming passion, and there is apparently no limit to what we will endure in the hope of losing weight. Even when it seems that the market must have reached saturation point, another "miracle diet" tops the bestseller list.

The Secret of Permanent Weight Loss

The sad truth, however, is that where diets are concerned, miracles don't exist. If they did, the problem of obesity would have been solved long ago and this book would not have been written. Let's be quite clear from the start: if a diet makes you eat less, it will also make you lose weight. Unfortunately, you won't lose it *permanently*. As soon as you come off the diet and begin to eat normally again, the weight creeps back and, before long, you are back where you started.

You cannot lose weight fast *and* lose it permanently. Any diet book that promises a slimmer figure within days should carry a sub-title guaranteeing the old one back in a matter of weeks. If this were just another of those books, you could stop reading right now. But it isn't. This book doesn't only tell you how to lose weight: it tells you how to put weight problems behind you forever, so that you can get on with enjoying life.

The Dancer's Diet

The idea of taking advice on diet from a ballet dancer might seem a little strange. After all, aren't dancers naturally blessed with perfect bodies? Surely they know nothing about struggling to control their weight? But think about it a little longer: you probably have two contrasting ideas about ballet dancers. The first is that we are all waif-like creatures who weigh less than our pointe shoes. The second is that we will happily go to horrific lengths in pursuit of what we call perfection.

Dancers, who in reality are of the same flesh and blood as everyone else, are usually fighting the same battle with their bodies. Until recently, I was no exception. Like many dancers, I have in the past had a rather "special" relationship with food. For the first twelve years of my professional life, I was in constant conflict with my body, struggling to maintain the sylph-like silhouette of a ballerina while still having enough energy to get up and dance. The two requirements did not seem compatible: I was born with the classic "pear" shape – hips wider than shoulders – and what seemed like an unconquerable tendency to gain weight. I tried every trick in the book (and some which are not) to combat this, in an endless cycle of yo-yo dieting – low-calorie, one-meal-a-day, near-starvation, and salad-and-fruit-only diets. I vainly hoped that by eating fewer calories than I needed, I would have no option but to burn the excess fat. Yet the only thing I consistently managed to lose was the energy I needed in my work. Some diets were more successful than others and, occasionally, the weight would drop off, but the end result was always the same: within a week or so, it was back.

Vital Statistics

I had almost given up the fight when I met Torje Eike

in 1993. With his expert knowledge of the way the

body works, he introduced me to a concept of eating

based on physiology: fact, rather than fiction. All my

previous convictions about diet were turned on their

head. For a long time I had avoided bread, pasta and

other forms of carbohydrates in the belief that they were

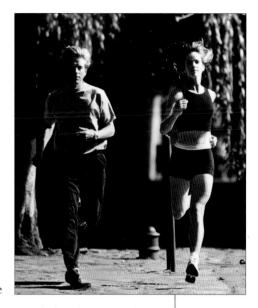

fattening, but Torje insisted that they were precisely the foods I should be eating –

they were the source of the energy I so badly needed. It was this connection between

food and fuel that started me on a journey of discovery. I gave up the search for a

magic formula for weight loss, and finally found what I was looking for in the

physiology of the human body itself.

Losing and controlling weight became no more than a question of accepting that the

body runs better on some fuels than others. If, like me, you thought dieting was

about self-deprivation, starvation and agonizing sessions in the gym, you're in for a

very pleasant surprise: losing weight is not about the things you should not do – it is

about the things you *should* do.

DEBORAH BULL

Weight Loss: The Facts

No matter how many failed diets we have under our belts, it is still
tempting to believe that there is, somewhere, a miracle diet that will help
us to shed pounds without any effort at all. I spent years searching for it, and
was taken in, time and time again, by the fresh and seductive promise of
a magic formula for weight loss.

Yet, however many diets I tried, I never managed to lose weight permanently.
It was only when I started to work with my body rather than fight against it,
that my personal battle became a thing of the past. It is the facts that provide
the answers and you need to understand those facts before weight control
makes sense. It may all seem a little complicated at first, but persevere:
battling with a few pages of information is going to
be a lot easier than battling against
your body.

The Myths

The human body is like a machine; it operates according to certain laws that cannot be ignored. Until I understood those laws, I tried every possible way to get thin, but failed with remarkable consistency: I had the will to succeed but lacked the knowledge. But before we face the facts, let's dispel a few myths.

1 The only way to lose weight is to eat less

It is unquestionably true that you can lose weight by eating less. Everyone has done it at some point, either through choice or illness. Depriving your body of the food it needs will undoubtedly lead to rapid loss of body mass. Whether it leads to rapid loss of *fat* is another matter. It is unlikely that there is any way, apart from surgery, that fat can be lost rapidly. Furthermore, scientific research proves that weight loss through diet alone is successful in the long term less than 20% of the time – in some studies it's even less.

2 The scales never lie

Unfortunately they do. Rapid weight loss looks so good on the scales because it is mainly a loss of water and muscle. Muscle, being compact, weighs much more than fat, so two people can weigh the same yet look very different. The best way to assess progress is to:
- Throw away your scales.
- Dig out an old pair of jeans that fitted when you were happy with your body. Try them on at regular intervals until you can fasten the zip.
- Congratulate yourself and keep going.

3 If I eat less than I need, my body will have to burn its excess fat

This would seem to be logical. We all have a lot of fat stored up and it is, in some circumstances, a very efficient source of energy. Unfortunately, not in this circumstance. Your body's first priority is always to protect the brain. The brain depends on glucose, from carbohydrates, for its fuel. Fat cannot be converted into glucose but, in emergencies, when no carbohydrates are available, protein can. When starved of food, the body turns to its protein stores to provide energy and you start to "eat" your own muscles.

4 Certain exercises burn fat from specific areas

The theory behind "spot reducing" is that muscle activity in a specific area stimulates the burning of the fat deposits closest to that muscle. So, to slim down your thighs, you cycle, or to flatten your stomach, you do sit-ups. Sadly, the body does not work like this. You cannot choose where you would like the fat to come from when you work out. Exercise stimulates a general rather than a specific use of fat, through hormones delivered in the bloodstream to the whole body. Exercise will, however, build lean tissue, which influences the metabolic rate (see Myth 8, opposite). Strengthening certain areas, such as the abdominals and the hamstrings, also improves posture and this in itself will have a positive effect on your appearance.

5 Some diets target weight from one body area, e.g. the hips

This idea could be part of Myth 4. Unfortunately, the theory doesn't add up and it is about as possible as emptying one side of a bottle.

6 Grapefruit and egg (substitute any food) is a magic combination for weight loss

"One-food-centred" diets are based on the idea that particular foods, or combinations of them, magically burn off fat. The theory is that the process of digesting certain foods requires more calories than they contain. You can lose weight fast on diets like these: they are very-low-calorie diets that border dangerously on starvation and you won't lose the weight permanently. Apart from being repetitious and boring, these diets seriously lack nutrients, slow down your metabolism and provide very little energy.

7 The body cannot digest certain foods at the same time

This "food combining" theory is based on the idea that the digestive enzymes that break down protein and carbohydrates neutralize each other, leaving undigested foods to ferment in the gut, become toxic and cause obesity and constipation. Medical opinion states that this type of diet only works because it makes the dieter monitor the quality and quantity of food they eat.

8 My metabolism is so slow I can't lose weight

Everyone claims to have a friend who "eats like a horse and never gains weight", but scientists are still looking for this person. Depending on age and gender, we all burn food at about the same rate. This is because our metabolic rate is linked to our lean tissue; women naturally have less muscle and more fat than men, and muscle tends to decrease with age. Muscle burns fuel faster than fat does because it is a working part of the body – fat is just something we carry around. Dramatic weight loss through dieting depletes muscle mass, lowering the metabolic rate. The body learns to survive on fewer calories and, after the diet, healthy amounts of food become surplus to requirements and are stored as fat. You regain weight quickly.

9 Wearing plastic or sweat gear helps weight loss

Forcing yourself to sweat makes you lose water, not fat. Water is essential to life and you can drink as much as you like – it contains no calories and no fat.

10 Exercise is a useless way to lose weight: you have to burn 3,500 calories to lose just 0.45kg/1lb of fat

It is true that 0.45kg (1lb) of fat is worth about 3,500 calories. If you are used to starvation diets, where the scales show a loss of five times this amount in a week, you might be disheartened. The only way you can lose that much "weight" in a week, however, is by losing muscle and water, and all the evidence shows it will very quickly return. Combining exercise with dieting means more of the weight lost will be fat. Remember, the scales don't tell the whole truth: muscle is heavier than fat. 0.45 kg (1lb) of fat takes up 508 cubic cm (31 cubic inches) of space – about the size of a cabbage. 0.45kg (1lb) of muscle only takes up 410 cubic cm (25 cubic inches). So, if you replaced 2.25kg (5lb) of fat with 2.25kg (5lb) of muscle, you would weigh the same but you would be around 492 cubic cm (30 cubic inches) smaller. Think about it.

The Facts

There is no secret formula for weight loss. You cannot lose weight without creating a "calorie deficit" – burning off more calories than you take in as food. In theory, you can choose one of three ways to do this: eat less, exercise more, or combine the two by eating a little less while exercising a little more. When the facts are laid out, the choice is obvious.

In contrast to all the myths about weight loss, there is one central fact:

Combining a reduced intake of food, that is high in carbohydrates and low in fat, with an appropriate exercise programme is the only way to lose body fat and lose it permanently.

A diet high in carbohydrates will give you plenty of energy to exercise. The benefits of exercise are twofold: it burns fat as a fuel and at the same time maintains muscle mass, so that your metabolic rate remains high, despite the fact that you are losing weight. It may not be as seductive as all those lose weight fast diets but it really is the closest you will ever get to a magic formula for permanent weight loss.

The practical method

No doctor would recommend that you lose more than about ½ – 1kg (about 1 – 2lb) of weight per week. 0.45kg (1lb) of fat represents approximately 3,500 calories. This may seem a vast amount of calories but, spread over a week, it averages out at no more than 500 calories per day. By combining the right type of exercise with the right type of diet, you can achieve this quite easily without either starving yourself or killing yourself in the gym.

It might seem like a slow process but you cannot lose weight quickly and lose it permanently. If you lose fat rather than muscle and water, you can be sure that the weight will stay off. Bear in mind that 0.45kg (1lb) of fat is equal to 508 cubic cm (31 cubic inches) of body mass, so over 10 weeks you could lose a massive 5,080 cubic cm (310 cubic inches) of fat. Now that is a lot of fat.

If you want to lose 0.45kg (1lb) of fat in a week, your calorie deficit should be 500 calories per day. You can achieve this by doing the following:

■ Decrease the energy you take in by 250 calories a day. Stick to foods that are high in carbohydrates and low in fat (see pages 38 – 39). Fat has over twice the calories of carbohydrates, so cutting down on fat is the simplest and healthiest way to reduce calories. Some carbohydrates release energy gradually, which keeps your blood-sugar level constant so you will not suffer from the sugar cravings, hunger and weakness that plague most attempts to lose weight.

■ At the same time, increase the energy you use every day by 250 calories. This is easily done with 30 minutes of moderate aerobic exercise, such as cycling or jogging, or with an hour's brisk walk. However unfit you feel, you can embark on an exercise programme that will build up safely to achieve this (see page 55).

The benefits of losing weight in this way are numerous:

High energy
A diet high in carbohydrates gives you maximum energy. In contrast, a low-calorie diet delivers exactly what it promises: low energy. A diet that makes you weak and hungry leaves you open to temptation, and usually results in bingeing, when the body's survival instinct takes over and does its best to persuade you to eat.

Weight loss is permanent
A diet high in carbohydrates provides plenty of energy to exercise, which helps to ensure that weight stays off. Quick-fix diets usually mean that you regain weight just as quickly as you lost it.

Body fat is substantially decreased
You can be sure that you are losing fat. Shorter periods of calorie restriction alone have been shown to result in temporary weight loss, mainly from muscle and water.

Exercise re-educates the body
If you exercise, your natural appetite cues are reprogrammed to respond to the need for food, while the appetite of an inactive person tends to "freewheel". A programme of weight loss that includes exercise relies less on reducing calories, so there is less hunger and less temptation.

Muscle mass is maintained
Aerobic exercise preserves muscle mass, while fat is burnt as a fuel, so your metabolic rate remains high.

Significant health benefits
Unique benefits are achieved by increasing exercise and reducing fat. These include a reduced risk of several obesity-linked diseases that can endanger the heart. Weight-bearing exercise also maintains bone mass and helps guard against osteoporosis in old age.

Exercise releases endorphins
These "feel-good" hormones give you an increased sense of wellbeing. Exercise also provides an outlet from the stresses of everyday life and a good work out will leave you feeling physically and mentally refreshed. You will also benefit from the positive feeling of actively contributing to your weight loss.

Using Energy

Muscles make up almost half of the body mass. There are over 660 different muscles in the human body and, even at rest, they account for about 20% of the average daily energy you use. During intense exercise, this can increase one hundredfold. The more exercise you do, the more energy the muscles burn.

Fuel for life

Although energy is usually associated with exercise, it is also used when you are at rest. Just as a car burns fuel even when the engine is idling, the body uses energy even when you are asleep, simply in order to stay alive. This energy is not conjured up from thin air: it comes from your daily diet. The food you eat goes through a digestive process in which the useful parts are extracted and the waste expelled. Anything beyond what you need gets stored for future use.

Storing energy

Muscles are made up of 75% protein and 20% water. They are dense and compact: 0.45kg (1lb) of muscle is 98 cubic cm (6 cubic inches) smaller in volume than 0.45kg (1lb) of fat. In the short term, a limited amount of carbohydrates can be stored in the muscles. The only long-term storage system the body has is fat. Its capacity to store fat is practically unlimited and it is the ultimate destination of any food that is surplus to requirements. The average person has 2,000 calories' worth of carbohydrates stored, compared to about 80,000 calories' worth of fat. That's enough carbohydrates to run 20 miles, and more than enough fat to run the length of Great Britain.

Burning fat: the problem

It may seem hard to believe, but the body actually prefers to use fat for energy. It likes to save the carbohydrates to feed the brain, which needs around 120g (4oz) daily – the sugar in ten apples. We worry, quite rightly, when the brain is starved of oxygen, yet people often go on diets that starve the brain of sugar.

The body has vast stores of fat available and wants to use them, so why is obesity such a problem? Firstly, it is because technology has eliminated most of the fat-burning activities from modern life; we can have clean clothes at the touch of a button and rarely walk anywhere. We're left with time on our hands and, as a direct consequence, flab on our hips. At the same time, food is cheaper and more plentiful than ever and we eat rich and fatty foods every day. We are simply eating more fat than we burn. The result is an alarming increase in obesity that is beginning to rival even smoking-related diseases as a cause of death.

The solution

The one method of weight control that is proven to be successful in the long term, works because it doesn't try to ignore the laws of nature. By combining a high-carbohydrate, low-fat diet with the right type of exercise, you can tackle both the major causes of obesity, so weight loss will be permanent. You can ignore all the "miracle" cures: when the facts are set out, you will find that they are too persuasive to ignore.

The Muscle Groups

Deltoid

Pectorals

Triceps

Biceps

Intercostals

Latissimus dorsi

Spinal column

Erector spinae

Rectus abdominis

Abdominal obliques

Psoas

Tensor fasciae latae

Gluteals

Rectus femoris

Adductors

Femur

Hamstrings

Gastrocnemius

Soleus

Diet or Exercise?

Most people who want to lose weight are more than willing to make whatever changes are necessary, but they aren't very clear on just what those changes should be. To lose weight in the long term, you have to consider diet, exercise and weight control as three connected points of the same triangle.

Understanding the connection

Almost everyone has an opinion on losing weight. Some say it doesn't matter how much exercise you do, it's cutting down what you eat that counts. Others swear that increasing your activity is the only way to make a difference: the harder you work, the more weight you lose. As you can see below, neither argument in itself gives you the whole picture.

Diet

You will lose weight if you consistently eat less food than your body needs, and it might look quite impressive on the scales.

But, diet without exercise makes you lose muscle and water, not fat, and within weeks the weight is bound to be back.

Exercise

Exercise is very effective at burning calories, and fat is a vast source of stored energy that can potentially be used as fuel.

However, if you continue to eat more fat than you need, the fat that you have lost will soon be back.

Weight control

*It has been proved repeatedly that, although you can lose weight through diet or exercise, the best way to reduce body fat **permanently** is to combine the right exercise (see opposite) with a low-fat, high-carbohydrate diet.*

The relationship between diet, exercise and weight control

What is Exercise?

Every weekend, the parks are full of "Sunday slimmers" attempting to sprint their way to a better figure. They go all out for as long as they can – a few minutes at the most – and are then forced to stop until they get their breath back again. They understand the need to exercise but they are going about it the wrong way.

The two types of exercise

"Exercise" can describe absolutely any physical activity, from walking the dog to running a marathon. Yet, however sedate or strenuous the exercise might be, the body only recognizes two types: "aerobic" and "anaerobic" exercise. Which type it is depends on two factors: intensity (how hard you work) and duration (how long the work lasts).

Intensity and duration

In short bursts, we can produce a considerable amount of power. Most of us can manage a fair pace if it means the difference between catching a bus or being forced to wait for the next one, and world-class sprinters can run the 400 metres in well under a minute. Yet, with all their years of training, even they can't continue at full speed for much longer than this. It is simply the way the human body works. We are not designed to keep up intense effort over a long period of time, and pushing the body to the limit means that we run out of steam quickly.

While a high degree of effort can be sustained in activity that lasts up to a minute or two, if the effort is reduced, we can keep up exercise for hours. We all know from experience that, whatever the activity, be it digging the garden or dancing the night away, the less effort we put in, the longer we can continue.

The length of time we can keep going during exercise is directly related to how hard we work. If exercise is so high in intensity that it limits duration, it is called "anaerobic" exercise, whereas if it is lower in intensity and sustainable, it is called "aerobic" exercise (see pages 20 – 21).

The effects of intensity vs duration

High

INTENSITY OF EXERCISE

Anaerobic energy

Anaerobic exercise involves high-intensity effort that can be sustained for only about a minute

Aerobic exercise can continue for several hours at low intensity

Aerobic energy

Low

0   1 minute   2 minutes   DURATION OF EXERCISE

What Type of Exercise?

Once you have accepted that exercise plays an important part in weight loss, you need to know what type of exercise you should do for it to have the most effect. To burn body fat, you must exercise at low to moderate intensity for at least 20 minutes.

The two energy systems

Just as there are two types of exercise, the body has two systems for producing the energy that exercise requires. These are called the anaerobic and aerobic systems. Both systems burn carbohydrates but only one of them, eventually, burns fat: unless your exercise is fuelled by the aerobic system, all the sweating in the world won't help. Very demanding exercise might keep you fit but it doesn't necessarily keep you thin.

The short-term (anaerobic) system

Anaerobic literally means "without air". During anaerobic exercise – intense exercise lasting about a minute – the demand for energy is either so sudden or so great that the heart is unable to pump enough oxygen to the working muscles.

Because there is insufficient oxygen in the muscles, the body has to find another way of producing energy – one that doesn't involve oxygen. It does this through a series of steps that break down carbohydrates to produce energy. All anaerobic exercise is fuelled by the anaerobic system, which burns carbohydrates, not fat. When you start to exercise, your heart begins to beat faster in response to the increased need for oxygen. Until enough oxygen becomes available to the muscles, all energy has to be supplied anaerobically. The anaerobic system therefore acts as the gateway to all activity, and the consequent build up of lactic acid (see side panel, left) explains the "heavy legs" that make exercise seem so tiring in the beginning. Once oxygen reaches the muscles, the lactic acid is recycled.

LACTIC ACID

The anaerobic system is sometimes known as the "lactic acid system". Lactic acid is blamed for sore muscles and cramp, and is seen as a waste product. In fact, it is vital to both the energy systems and is formed even when we rest. It is only a problem during anaerobic exercise, when it builds up in the muscles until we are forced to ease off or stop.

ANAEROBIC EXERCISE

High intensity, short duration

- *Running up the stairs*
- *Sprinting*
- *Push-starting the car*

The long-term (aerobic) system

Aerobic means "with air". All oxygen is delivered around the body in blood pumped by the heart. The aerobic system can function only when the energy demand is low enough for the heart to supply the muscles with sufficient oxygen – the sort of exercise when you are breathing hard, but not gasping for breath.

Aerobic exercise is predominantly fuelled by the aerobic system. Both carbohydrates and fat can supply fuel for this system but, when exercise lasts for less than 20 minutes, carbohydrates will always provide the fuel. Only when the exercise goes beyond this, can fat contribute to the supply.

AEROBIC EXERCISE

Low to moderate intensity, long duration

- *Walking the dog*
- *Jogging*
- *Cycling to the shops*

☐ Anaerobic exercise

☐ Aerobic exercise

☐ Aerobic endurance exercise

Aerobic endurance

There is a variation of aerobic exercise called "aerobic endurance exercise". This is when exercise continues at a low level over a long period of time. *It is only during this type of activity that fat is broken down and used as the main source of energy.*

Fat molecules are difficult to break down, and it takes the body a while to "gear up" its fat-burning cycle. This is why exercise designed specifically to burn fat is sometimes called "endurance" exercise. Unless your work out is relatively low in intensity and lasts over 20 minutes, the body has no choice but to burn stored carbohydrates instead. While carbohydrates can fuel both energy systems, fat can only be burnt in aerobic endurance exercise. If you want to get rid of excess body fat once and for all, this type of exercise is, without a doubt, the best way to do it. Although 20 minutes' or more exercise may sound like a lot, don't be put off. The whole point of aerobic endurance exercise is that the intensity is low enough to be easily sustained over a long period of time.

Fat doesn't fuel all long-term exercise. When high-intensity exercise continues over a long time, carbohydrates provide the energy, so marathon runners are fuelled primarily by the pasta they eat in the days before the race. You can store enough carbohydrates to provide the energy for about 90 minutes of high-intensity exercise. As there are several endurance events that last longer than this, there is a time when carbohydrate stores will run out; this is commonly known as "hitting the wall". Neither energy process happens independently of the other, and they can and do overlap. The body switches between the systems according to the demands you make of it.

LIMITED LUNG CAPACITY

Every healthy person can do aerobic endurance exercise. Some people use "limited lung capacity" as an excuse if they get seriously out of breath, but the limiting factor here is usually their heart's inefficiency through lack of exercise. The heart is a muscle which, like any other, can be improved with training. An individual's lung capacity is more or less fixed.

AEROBIC ENDURANCE EXERCISE

Low intensity, over 20-minutes' duration

- *An hour's walk*
- *30 minutes of cycling*
- *A country hike*

Reading Your Heart Rate

If you want to lose body fat permanently, you have to use it as a fuel in aerobic endurance exercise (see page 21). Your watch tells you how long you are working – the endurance element – and it can also help you check that you aren't working too hard.

Hitting the right intensity

You find out how hard you are working by measuring your heart rate. During exercise, your heart rate goes up; the harder you work, the faster the heart beats. Everyone has a maximum heart rate – the fastest it can possibly beat. Calculating how close your heart rate is to its maximum during exercise enables you to check the intensity of your work out.

Reading your heart rate

Your training heart rate must be measured during exercise, but you may find it useful to take a few practice readings while resting. It takes time to become proficient and initial attempts may be a little far-fetched.

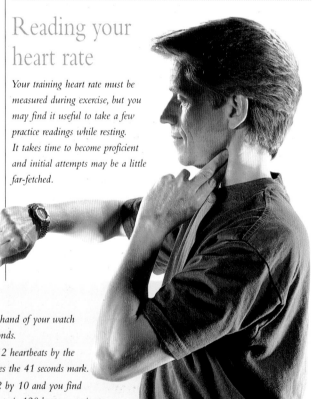

1 *Find your pulse either on the underside of your wrist, or on the side of your neck. Use your first two fingers, not the thumb, as it has its own pulse which can distort the accuracy of a reading. You may need to make a brief stop, but take your pulse immediately.*

2 *Start counting your pulse when the second hand of your watch reaches a given point, and count the beats over the next six seconds.*

3 *Multiply this number by 10 to work out the number of beats in 60 seconds and you have the beats per minute (BPM). This is your heart rate. You can test the accuracy by counting the beats over 30 seconds and multiplying them by 2 to see if you get the same result.*

EXAMPLE

- *The second hand of your watch is at 35 seconds.*
- *You count 12 heartbeats by the time it reaches the 41 seconds mark.*
- *Multiply 12 by 10 and you find your heart rate is 120 beats per minute.*

Using a heart-rate monitor

You can also check your heart rate using an electronic heart-rate monitor. This will give an accurate read-out of your heart rate throughout exercise. Different models are available but you only need the most basic (and the cheapest).

1 *Strap the transmitter band of the monitor around your chest, directly next to your skin. This will relay information to the monitor.*

2 *Strap the monitor, which resembles a digital watch, to your wrist. The display will show you a constant reading of your heart rate.*

Your maximum heart rate

To calculate if you are working at the right intensity, you also need to know your maximum heart rate. Although there are tests to measure this, they aren't necessary unless you have a heart problem; instead, it can be estimated. As you get older, the maximum rate at which your heart can beat decreases, so the age-based formula on the right works as a guideline.

Your age-predicted maximum heart rate = (220 - your age)

- *If you are 18 years old, your age-predicted maximum will be:*   *220 - 18 = 202 BPM*
- *If you are 25 years old:*   *220 - 25 = 195 BPM*
- *If you are 35 years old:*   *220 - 35 = 185 BPM*
- *If you are 50 years old:*   *220 - 50 = 170 BPM*
- *If you are 65 years old:*   *220 - 65 = 155 BPM*

Target zones for different types of exercise

In anaerobic exercise	In aerobic exercise	In aerobic endurance exercise
Your heart is working faster than 85% of its maximum heart rate (see above):	Your heart is working between 60% and 85% of its maximum heart rate (see above):	Your heart is working between 60% and 70% of its maximum heart rate (see above) for at least 20 minutes:
Running up the stairs	Walking the dog	An hour's walk
Sprinting	Jogging	30 minutes of cycling
Push-starting the car	Cycling to the shops	A country hike
■ If you are 18 years old: at least **171 BPM**	■ If you are 18 years old: between **121** and **171 BPM**	■ If you are 18 years old: between **121** and **141 BPM**
■ If you are 25 years old: at least **165 BPM**	■ If you are 25 years old: between **117** and **165 BPM**	■ If you are 25 years old: between **117** and **136 BPM**
■ If you are 35 years old: at least **157 BPM**	■ If you are 35 years old: between **111** and **157 BPM**	■ If you are 35 years old: between **111** and **129 BPM**
■ If you are 50 years old: at least **144 BPM**	■ If you are 50 years old: between **102** and **144 BPM**	■ If you are 50 years old: between **102** and **119 BPM**
■ If you are 65 years old: at least **131 BPM**	■ If you are 65 years old: between **93** and **131 BPM**	■ If you are 65 years old: between **93** and **108 BPM**

CAUTION

If you have a family history of heart problems, check with your GP before starting any exercise programme.

Energy for Life

Total Nutrition Guide

Most of us have, at some time in our lives, suffered the hunger

pangs that come with a "low-calorie diet" yet, despite all the

effort it involves, dieting is usually a short-term solution to a

long-term problem. Sustained, healthy weight control lies

in finding the right balance between the different types

of food you eat.

But how can you translate this theory to the food on your plate?

Traditional diets rely on obsessively counting calories, yet there is a

much simpler way. Understanding the essentials of healthy eating

was, for me, the key to controlling my weight without losing

energy, and I haven't felt hungry since.

The Low-down on Calories

For most people, "going on a diet" means counting and cutting calories. Filled with optimism and determination, they clear the fridge of anything vaguely appetizing and load it up with foods that boast they "help slimming as part of a calorie-controlled diet".

What is a calorie?

You can certainly lose weight on a calorie-controlled diet, although for how long is open to question. Unfortunately, you'll also lose the most important thing that calories supply: energy. Despite years of obsessively counting them, most dieters are still not very clear on exactly what a calorie is. Before you decide to cut them, it might be a good idea to find out.

Cutting energy

Most of the food you buy (and certainly all the packaged food) tells you how many calories it contains. You'll find it listed under one of three words: "kcals", "kjoules" or "energy". The last of these provides the clue. The calorific content of food doesn't indicate how fat you'll get if you eat that food; it tells you how much energy it will provide. This is why cutting calories inevitably means cutting energy; the two words are interchangeable. In nutritional terms, calories measure the energy provided by the food you eat to "heat" or fuel your body. "Calorific expenditure" is the amount of energy you use.

If that was the end of the story, you could argue that the more calories you eat, the more energy you have and, in a way, you would be right. You would certainly have a lot of potential energy, but recent research shows that you would be unlikely to use it. We burn far fewer calories every week than our grandparents did, and our lifestyles rarely include the sort of long-term activity that burns fat. Most of the energy we use comes from carbohydrates. Unfortunately, less useful calories don't just disappear. You either use them or you store them, and the only long-term storage system we have is body fat.

Where do calories come from?

With one exception, calories come from three sources: carbohydrates, protein and fat provide all the energy, and therefore the calories, your body needs, but the recipe for good health has three other essential ingredients: vitamins, minerals and water. The absence of any one of these six elements would eventually lead to illness and, in the long term, would prove fatal. Vitamins, minerals and water play an important part in just about everything that goes on in the body but, contrary to popular belief, they do not supply energy; they are calorie-free, and energy comes only with calories.

Alcohol also supplies a considerable number of calories but it contributes very little to sound nutrition. If you're trying to lose weight, you should try to drink as little alcohol as possible.

Although most food can be categorized as predominantly carbohydrates, protein or fat, there are very few that are made up of only one of these. In most cases, the calories come from two or three sources. To control your weight, it's not the number of calories you should be watching, but where they come from. Some calories are just more useful than others.

How many calories do you need?

Your body uses energy simply to stay alive. The resting metabolic rate tells you how many calories your body would use if you spent the entire day lying down. To get an idea of how much energy you really use, you have to add on the energy required in day-to-day living – getting up and going to work, for instance – and the energy you use in eating and digesting food. These three elements make up your total daily energy expenditure.

Survival tactics

It is highly unlikely that, as an adult, your body can maintain itself on fewer than 1,200 calories a day. If you try to survive on less than this, you will be hard-pushed to get all the nutrients you require for long-term health. In addition, taking in fewer calories than your body needs encourages it to break down protein (your muscles) to supply energy. As they influence your metabolism, depleting the muscles leads to a lowering of your metabolic rate.

Dramatic weight loss through diet alone has been proven to have a serious and sustained effect on the metabolism, above and beyond the effect of losing lean tissue. The body is designed to survive famine, even if it is self-inflicted. In severe diets, the metabolic rate can be depressed by as much as 45% as the body becomes more "energy efficient", slowing down its systems to enable it to survive on fewer calories. It's a bit like driving a car which is low on petrol. If you want to make it last until the nearest garage, you have no option but to drive very slowly. The lower the speed, the less fuel you burn. As your metabolic rate goes down, the body uses less energy, and you will find it harder to lose weight, however little you eat. Regular exercise, on the other hand, can raise your metabolic rate by maintaining, and even increasing, muscle mass.

ESTIMATING YOUR RESTING METABOLIC RATE (RMR)

You can estimate your RMR by multiplying your weight in pounds by 10 (1lb = 0.45kg)

- *If you weigh 130lb, your RMR will be approximately 1,300 calories: 130 X 10 = 1,300*

Remember, the resting metabolic rate is not your ideal calorie intake; it only tells you how many calories you would use to lie in bed all day.

How the body uses energy

Between 60 – 75 % of the energy you use in a day is taken up in staying alive. Physical activity – working, shopping or exercising – accounts for a further 15 – 30%, depending on how active you are, and a small amount of energy is used to digest food. By far the easiest way to increase your energy expenditure is to add on exercise; builders and endurance athletes can use twice as much energy every day as the average adult.

RESTING METABOLIC RATE USES 60 – 75% OF TOTAL DAILY ENERGY

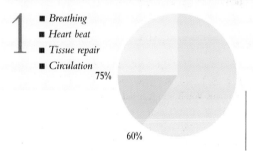

1
- Breathing
- Heart beat
- Tissue repair
- Circulation

75%

60%

PHYSICAL ACTIVITY USES 15 – 30% OF TOTAL DAILY ENERGY

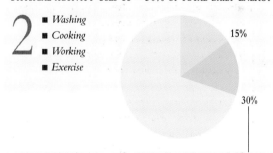

2
- Washing
- Cooking
- Working
- Exercise

15%

30%

EATING AND DIGESTING FOOD USES 10% OF TOTAL DAILY ENERGY

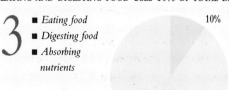

3
- Eating food
- Digesting food
- Absorbing nutrients

10%

Carbohydrates

This is a catch-all term for starchy and sweet foods, from pasta to sugar lumps. Carbohydrates are the major fuel for all physical activity – not just the kind of exercise that athletes do, but running for the bus as well. A low-carbohydrate diet leads to low energy, which leads to low activity – this is how weight creeps up.

What do they do?

- Stored in the liver and muscles as glycogen, carbohydrates serve as a major energy source for all activity.
- Carbohydrates are the main fuel of the central nervous system, which includes the brain.
- They are an essential part of the fat-burning process and serve as a "primer": if carbohydrates are not present, fat cannot be broken down completely.
- They provide 4 calories of energy per gram.

Where are they found?

Nature has given us three types of carbohydrates, all of which can be called "unrefined".

"Simple" carbohydrates

Often referred to collectively as "simple sugars", these include: glucose (a sugar that occurs naturally in foods such as fruit), fructose (another natural sugar in fruit), lactose (present in milk, including breast milk) and sucrose (found in sugar cane).

"Complex" carbohydrates

These are also known as starches. Plants store carbohydrates as starch, and it is found in rice, flour and potatoes. Starch is made up of a chain of simple sugars that are linked together, so it is slower to break down and releases its energy over a longer period.

GOOD SOURCES OF
UNREFINED
CARBOHYDRATES

Choose wholegrain
varieties whenever
possible.

■

PASTA

■

BREAD

■

BREAKFAST CEREALS

■

GRAINS, SUCH AS RICE,
COUSCOUS, WHEAT,
FLOUR

■

BEANS

■

FRUIT

■

DRIED FRUIT

■

POTATOES AND OTHER
ROOT VEGETABLES

DAILY REQUIREMENT

Unrefined
carbohydrate foods
should make up
more than 50%
of the food
on your plate.

Dietary fibre

An integral part of most unrefined carbohydrates, fibre is found in the cell walls of vegetables, fruit, beans and wholegrain cereals. Most fibre cannot be digested by humans but it is still extremely beneficial. It provides bulk that makes you feel full and naturally limits the amount you eat at any one time. Fibre also acts as a binding agent and speeds up the passage of food through the intestines. In this way, fibre helps to guard against gastrointestinal disease and colon cancer.

Refined sugar

Man has managed to introduce a fourth carbohydrate into the diet. Refined sugar, such as table sugar, is not found in nature, which is a good indication of just how much your body needs it. It is used to add sweetness to confectionery, cakes, biscuits and a good deal of supposedly savoury food. It provides plenty of calories and therefore plenty of energy, but contributes no nutritional value to your diet, as refined carbohydrates are stripped of all their vitamins, minerals and fibre. Refined sugar releases its energy very quickly, triggering an abrupt insulin response that can lead to light-headedness and "blood sugar jitters" (see page 54). After an initial high, your energy levels will feel lower than they did before you ate, until they eventually stabilize.

Unrefined vs refined carbohydrates

Unrefined carbohydrates, such as wholemeal bread, wholewheat pasta, wholegrain cereals, brown rice and fruit, provide valuable vitamins and minerals along with energy. The process of refining wholewheat flour into white flour, for example, strips it of nutrients, leaving little else apart from calories. This is one of the reasons why unrefined carbohydrates are a much healthier choice.

Weight control

As well as providing vitamins and minerals, unrefined carbohydrates contribute fibre to the diet, which is an important factor in appetite control (and in curbing weight gain). I find it impossible to overeat on unrefined carbohydrates – they are almost self-limiting. You feel full much sooner after a meal of unrefined carbohydrates than after one based on protein, fat or refined sugar, so you can satisfy your appetite without overloading on calories. A jacket potato, for example, has the same amount of energy/calories as an iced doughnut but, whereas a doughnut is mainly sugar and fat, a potato is high in fibre and complex carbohydrates. You might be able to eat two or three doughnuts, but you would be hard-pushed to manage more than one large baked potato. Foods high in unrefined carbohydrates are not only more filling, they are also usually lower in fat.

CARBOHYDRATE FOODS TO LIMIT IN YOUR DIET

- SUGAR (WHITE & BROWN)
- SWEETS
- CHOCOLATE
- CAKES
- SWEET BISCUITS
- SUGARY DRINKS
- JAM
- HONEY
- SYRUPS

Protein

The role of protein – maintaining and repairing tissue – cannot be fulfilled by any other nutrient, but there is no benefit at all from eating excessive amounts. Protein won't give you more energy or stronger muscles and it can be detrimental rather than beneficial to health.

In fact, you need much less protein than you may imagine.

**LOW-FAT SOURCES
OF PROTEIN**

Remove the fat or
skin from meat and
poultry, and use a
low-fat method of
cooking, such as
steaming or grilling,
to prepare food.

■

VERY LEAN MEAT

■

FISH

■

SKINLESS POULTRY

■

TOFU

■

PEAS & BEANS

■

LOW-FAT DAIRY
PRODUCTS

■

SMALL AMOUNTS
OF PROTEIN ARE
ALSO FOUND IN
BREAD, PASTA &
BREAKFAST CEREALS

What does it do?

■ Protein maintains, repairs and builds the living tissue in the body but, contrary to popular opinion, you don't increase muscle bulk by eating extra protein.
■ It is the main component of muscles, tendons and ligaments.
■ Protein can be converted to glucose and can provide energy for both the muscles and the brain when you eat insufficient amounts of carbohydrates. The use of protein for energy will take precedence over its foremost task of maintaining tissues, which means injuries and wounds will be slow to heal.
■ Protein provides 4 calories of energy per gram.

Where is it found?

Protein is present in most foods. It is made up of several amino acids, the building blocks of living tissue. You need around 20 different amino acids and they can be split into two categories. Eight of them (nine for children) cannot be made within the body, so you have to get them from what you eat. They are known as "essential" amino acids. This does not mean that the remaining twelve are not necessary – they are all vital for health, but the others can be manufactured in the body from the essential amino acids in your diet.

Protein quality

Foods contain amino acids in varying proportions and the quality of a protein is measured by how closely the amino acids match the human body's requirements. The closer the match, the more efficiently it can be used. The amino acids in animal proteins, such as eggs, milk, cheese, meat, poultry and fish, are very similar to human requirements. They are said to have a high "biological value", and may be described as "complete" proteins. Protein from plant sources is not generally as well-matched but, as meals are usually based around a variety of foods

DAILY REQUIREMENT

Protein should make
up 10 – 20% of the
daily diet.

such as bread with cheese, rice with lentils, or vegetables with pasta, it is not difficult to get a well-balanced mix of amino acids, even if you don't eat meat. You don't need to balance the amino acids in every meal, but the greater the variety of protein sources in your diet, the better.

The best sources of protein

Protein is present, to some degree, in almost everything you eat; the only foods that contain absolutely no protein are vegetable and nut oils, and refined table sugar. Protein is not particularly high in most fruit and vegetables, although foods from other plant sources, such as beans, wholegrain cereals, rice and pasta, contain a significant amount of it. Vegetarians and vegans who eat a wide variety of these foods should not be protein-deficient, especially if they eat soya beans, which are as high in protein as eggs and cheese.

The great protein myth

Despite the wealth of sensible information that is available, there is a persistent misunderstanding about protein and how much is really needed: ideally, it should only make up between 10 – 20% of what you eat.

Since the heyday of the high-protein/low-carbohydrate diet in the Seventies, grilled steak and lean chicken have been the cornerstone of the slimmer's diet. Potatoes and pasta continue to be seen as no-go areas for anyone watching their weight yet, while many high-carbohydrate foods contain only a trace of fat, high-protein foods are often a source of hidden fat. Even lean beef derives about 50% of its calories from fat, and the other 50% from protein. Although protein is certainly an important part of the diet – we couldn't function without it – according to recent US research, when the most popular types of diet were compared, the high-protein/low-carbohydrate diet was the only one for which no advantages could be found.

In a high-protein regime, when you restrict the amount of carbohydrates you eat, the body is forced to use protein as an energy source. The stores of carbohydrates (about 2,000 calories' worth) are used up in about 24 hours. The brain needs a constant level of sugar in the blood and, when it isn't provided in the diet, the body supplies it by converting protein into glucose. This diverts protein from its main task of repairing and maintaining tissue. In extreme cases of starvation, the body turns to its protein stores, the muscles, to provide energy. Losing muscle mass through dieting can lead to a lowering of the metabolic rate and can be dangerous.

Weight control

Today, 70% of the protein we eat is derived from animal produce; seventy years ago, it came equally from plants and animals. As meat products contain not only protein but also fat, many of us are eating much higher levels of saturated fat than we need. It is hardly surprising that up to a quarter of adults in the Western world are considered overweight and that heart disease is now a major cause of death in most industrialized nations.

HIGH-FAT SOURCE
OF PROTEIN

FATTY MEAT

EGGS

FULL-FAT DAIRY
PRODUCTS

NUTS

Fat

As much as everyone loves to hate it, fat is suprisingly palatable; it adds flavour and texture to the food we eat. A little fat is vital for good health, but as fat is present in most foods, especially those high in protein, it creeps into your diet more than you realize. Unless you eat a very limited diet, you should get enough fat without trying.

SOURCES OF UNSATURATED FAT

- VEGETABLE OILS
- OLIVE OIL
- NUT OILS
- AVOCADO
- NUTS
- SEEDS
- OILY FISH, SUCH AS TUNA, HERRING MACKEREL & SARDINES

What does it do?

- Certain fatty acids are essential: they cannot be made in the body yet are needed to help form cell walls and for growth, sexual reproduction and skin maintenance.
- The fat-soluble vitamins A, D, E and K are carried in fat.
- Fat is important as a fuel in light and moderate long-term activity.
- At 9 calories per gram, fat provides over twice as much energy as carbohydrates.

Where is it found?

There are two types of fat: saturated and unsaturated. Unsaturated fat is no lower in calories than any other fat, but it's a better choice, as saturated fat can raise blood cholesterol levels which can lead to heart disease. For good health, at least two-thirds of the fat you eat should be unsaturated.

Saturated fat

Found mainly in animal and dairy products, like butter, lard, cheese, fatty meat, eggs and whole milk, saturated fat tends to be solid at room temperature: the firmer the fat, the more saturated it is. There are some exceptions to this – palm and coconut oil are high in saturated fat, despite being liquid.

Unsaturated fat

There are two types of unsaturated fat: polyunsaturated and monounsaturated, and they are usually liquid at room temperature. Olive oil is probably the best-known source of monounsaturated fat; other sources include rapeseed oil and sesame oil. Polyunsaturated fat includes sunflower oil, soya oil, safflower oil, corn oil, walnut oil, peanut oil and fish oil. Replacing saturated with unsaturated fat can reduce the level of LDL, or "bad", cholesterol, the type that leads to narrowing of the arteries. The omega-3 fatty acids found in cold-water fish, such as tuna, herring, mackerel and sardines, are thought to have a beneficial effect on health, lowering the risk of heart disease.

DAILY REQUIREMENT

Fat should make up no more than 30% of your diet. If you are trying to lose weight, you may want to eat even less.

Hydrogenated fat

Most margarines and spreads contain a mixture of fats, yet advertize that they are "high in polyunsaturates". The process of hydrogenation makes liquid fats solid enough to be sold in a tub rather than a bottle. It adds hydrogen, which converts unsaturated fat into saturated fat, making it less beneficial to health. Hydrogenated fat is also found in foods such as sausages, pies, biscuits and cakes.

Cholesterol

A vital substance in the body, cholesterol is made by all animals, including humans. If your diet is high in saturated fat, the liver is stimulated to make more cholesterol than the body needs. The level of cholesterol in the blood goes up, and cholesterol-rich deposits are formed in the arteries which supply the heart with blood. This causes them to narrow, and can eventually lead to a heart attack. Saturated fat has a more harmful effect than the cholesterol found in foods, but substituting unsaturated fats can help to lower blood cholesterol levels. Cholesterol is not found in plant foods.

Lowering your fat intake

There are two major reasons why you should keep the fat you eat to a minimum: it is bad for your health, and it leads to weight gain. Any excess food you eat will be stored as body fat, however, fat is more easily converted to body fat than any other nutrient. The best way to lose weight is to replace fat with carbohydrate-rich foods and many foods are now available in reduced or low-fat versions. Some stores highlight items that are naturally low in fat but, beware, when fat is removed or reduced, it is often (not always) replaced with refined sugar. The list below gives alternatives that are no less filling, but that are much less fattening:

**SOURCES OF
SATURATED FAT**

FATTY CUTS OF MEAT

MEAT PRODUCTS, SUCH
AS SAUSAGES & PIES

FULL-FAT DAIRY
PRODUCTS

BUTTER

SOME MARGARINES

PALM OIL

COCONUT OIL

BISCUITS

CAKES

SAVOURY SNACKS

CUT OUT	REPLACE WITH
▪ Croissants	Low-fat bagels
▪ Butter or margarine	Low-fat spread
▪ Full-fat dairy products	Low-fat dairy products
▪ Cream- or oil-based salad dressings	Yoghurt-based or low-fat dressings
▪ Chips	Potatoes, boiled or baked
▪ Cheese or cream sauces	Vegetable-based sauces
▪ Fried fish or meat	Grilled fish or meat
▪ Fatty meat, sausages or pies	Poultry without skin, lean cuts of meat
▪ Sweets, snacks and crisps	Fruit, rice cakes, vegetables

Vitamins & Minerals

An essential part of every process that happens in the body, these nutrients are vital for good health. Supplements are rarely necessary, as a varied diet normally provides all you need.

GOOD SOURCES OF VITAMINS & MINERALS

RAW FRUIT & VEGETABLES

LIGHTLY COOKED, FRESH OR FROZEN FRUIT & VEGETABLES

WHOLEGRAIN CEREALS & GRAINS

LOW-FAT DAIRY PRODUCTS

BEANS & PEAS

LEAN MEAT

DAILY REQUIREMENT
Eat five or more different fruit and vegetables each day to ensure a good intake of vitamins and minerals. Choose fresh or frozen in preference to canned (see pages 38 – 39).

What do they do?

■ There are 13 known vitamins which play a vital role in most body processes. Whatever the adverts say, vitamins and minerals do not supply energy, they only assist in the release of it.

■ There are 22 known minerals which regulate body functions and provide structure in the formation of bones and teeth.

Where are they found?

As the body cannot manufacture vitamins or minerals, these nutrients must be included in your diet. Vitamins are found in all fresh, raw food, but processing, over-cooking, or storing food for long periods of time, reduces the vitamin content. Lightly cooked food (steamed or grilled) is the best option. You need vitamins in very small amounts, and it is much better to get them as part of a healthy diet than through expensive supplements. Most minerals occur freely in nature: in water, topsoil and below the earth's surface. They are therefore found in the plants and animals you eat and a varied, balanced diet should provide all the minerals you need.

Vitamins

There are two types of vitamins. Fat-soluble vitamins – A, D, E and K – are stored in the body for long periods of time, so it takes months of deprivation before deficiency becomes a problem. Water-soluble vitamins – B complex and C – cannot be stored and must be included in your daily diet. Any excess is usually excreted in urine, although some can accumulate in the body. A balanced diet should provide all the vitamins you need. If you think you need a supplement, limit yourself to a multi-vitamin that provides the recommended daily amount. Diagnosing individual vitamin deficiencies is best left to your doctor, as overdoses can be toxic.

Minerals

A balanced diet should provide you with sufficient minerals, but you should pay particular attention to your intake of calcium and iron.

Calcium Vital for nerve transmission and blood clotting, calcium also gives bones their strength. If you do not eat sufficient calcium, the body steals it from the bones. This can lead to osteoporosis, a condition that makes the bones fragile and prone to fracture. Osteoporosis does affect men, however, women are at greater risk, especially if they are very thin, eat insufficient calcium-rich foods, drink too much caffeine, or smoke. The female hormone oestrogen, which has a protective effect on bone-mass, is reduced after the menopause. Women who do not menstruate regularly are also particularly vulnerable and should consult a doctor. The best defence against osteoporosis is to combine a good calcium intake with weight-bearing exercise, such as brisk walking, which stimulates bone formation. Women should try to maximize bone strength during their twenties.

Sources: Milk, dairy produce (low-fat versions contain just as much), sardines and canned salmon (as long as you eat the bones), tofu, green leafy vegetables and beans. You need about 800mg of calcium a day.

Iron As this mineral is lost during menstruation, iron deficiency is fairly common in women. This is one of the few instances when a doctor may prescribe a supplement.
Sources: Red meat, liver, egg yolk, green leafy vegetables, bread, beans, fortified breakfast cereal and some dried fruit. The iron in non-meat produce is not as well-absorbed by the body, but you can increase its absorption by eating or drinking a source of vitamin C, such as a glass of orange juice, at the same time. A simple way to increase iron intake is to cook with unenamelled, cast-iron saucepans.

Salt Sweating causes the body to lose salt, but the need for added salt is probably more imagined than real. Most of us eat twice as much salt as we need. Excess sodium (a component of salt) can lead to high blood pressure, which in turn can increase the risk of strokes.
Sources: Watch out for added salt in smoked fish, savoury snacks and in many processed foods.

FOODS WITH A REDUCED VITAMIN & MINERAL CONTENT

■

FOOD STORED FOR A LONG TIME

■

OVER-COOKED FOOD

■

FOOD KEPT WARM FOR A LONG TIME

■

CANNED FOOD

■

PROCESSED FOOD

■

PEELED FRUIT & VEGETABLES

■

REFINED FOOD

Water

Of the six components necessary for a healthy diet, water is probably the most overlooked. It contains no carbohydrates, protein or fat and therefore no calories, yet it is crucial for survival.

DRINKS THAT
HYDRATE

■

WATER

■

FRUIT JUICE

■

HERB TEAS

■

FRUIT TEAS

■

SKIMMED &
SEMI-SKIMMED MILK

What does it do?

■ It transports nutrients into and throughout the body, and carries waste products out again.
■ Body temperature is stabilized by water.
■ Water is essential for lubricating the joints, and also helps blood and other tissue fluids to flow freely.

Where is it found ?

Most of your daily intake of water is from drinks, but a significant amount is provided by food. Some foods, such as fruit and vegetables, contain a great deal of water: bananas, for example, are 75% water. In contrast, other foods, like butter, oil, biscuits and cakes, contain very little. A small amount of water is also produced by the body during the process of breaking down food for energy.

Tea, coffee and most canned fizzy drinks contain caffeine, which is a diuretic and speeds up the loss of water, increasing dehydration. Drinks that are high in sugar aren't much help either, as sugar slows down the rate at which water can be absorbed from the stomach and put to use. Even fruit juices can be deceptively high in sugar. The most efficient drink for quenching thirst is also the most straightforward: cool, preferably not iced, water.

Fluid balance

You can last without food for several weeks, but you can't survive for more than a few days without water. The amount of water you drink should balance the amount you use. An adult needs about 2.5 litres (4 pints) – around eight glasses – of water a day; in hot weather, or during exercise, you obviously need more.

Despite its importance, very few people drink enough water. By the time you feel thirsty, the dehydration process is already well under way and reaching for a drink that dehydrates makes the situation worse.

DAILY REQUIREMENT

An adult needs about 2.5 litres (4 pints) of water a day. For every 30 minutes of exercise, you should drink a glass of water.

Water loss

Water is lost from the body in several ways:

As urine When protein is broken down, it leaves a waste product, called urea, that must be expelled from the body in urine. The more protein you eat, the more urea you produce. As more water is then needed to flush away the urea, if you eat large quantities of protein it can speed up dehydration.

As faeces This is made up of approximately 70% water, and accounts for a loss of about 100ml (4fl oz) of water a day. Diarrhoea or vomiting can increase the fluid loss to 5 litres (8 pints) and fluid replacement is vital.

Through the skin To maintain body temperature, you continually lose a small amount of fluid through your skin, called insensible perspiration, without ever being aware of it. You also lose over 600ml (1 pint) of water every day in sweat – exercising in hot climates can produce up to 1 litre (1.75 pints) of sweat an hour.

From the lungs When you exhale, water is lost. You only see it in very cold weather, when your breath forms a mist, but it is there whatever the temperature.

Losing water vs losing weight

Water accounts for about two-thirds of your body weight. Getting rid of this water by sweating might seem like a good way to lose weight, but losing water is not the same as losing fat: if it were, the clothes you sweat in would feel greasy, not wet.

If you stand on the scales as soon as you finish a sweaty work out, weight loss will seem to have occurred. But wait a few hours, drink a glass or two of water, and weigh yourself again: you will find that your weight is pretty much back to normal. It isn't a good idea to try to sweat yourself thin. Firstly, it won't work as any weight loss will only be temporary and, more importantly, losing even a small amount of water has serious health implications. It can affect blood pressure, temperature regulation and co-ordination and, when co-ordination is impaired, you are at risk of injury.

It is not sweat itself, but the evaporation of sweat that is the cooling mechanism of the body. In 100% humidity, the air is already saturated with as much water as it can hold, and sweat cannot evaporate. It simply rolls off the body and the cooling effect is lost.

Wearing plastic (sweat or sauna) pants affects the efficiency of sweating. By preventing the evaporation of sweat, plastic pants simply inhibit your cooling system and your body overheats. Body wraps in beauty salons work on the same principle; despite the miraculous claims for weight loss, the only thing you are losing is fluid. As soon as the body's water levels are replenished, you return to your original weight. Water loss doesn't affect body fat one little bit.

DRINKS THAT DEHYDRATE

Drinks that contain caffeine

∎

COFFEE

∎

TEA

∎

COLA

∎

SOME ENERGY DRINKS

Striking a Balance

The secret of long-term weight loss does not lie in counting calories; it lies in striking a balance by making sure that the different types of food on your plate are there in the right proportions. You should get more of your calories from high-carbohydrate foods and fewer from fat.

The right balance

No diet in the world would tell you to eat as much as you like and still lose weight – if you find one that does, ignore it. There have to be a few guidelines, but these do not have to be too harsh or extreme. A diet will not work if you cannot keep it up in the long term.

A high-carbohydrate, low-fat diet provides energy and nutrients without overloading on calories but, as very few foods are 100% carbohydrates, protein or fat, you have to learn to recognize what different foods are made of, and mix and match them to create a diet that follows these guidelines:

Eat unlimited

Eat a good selection of at least five types of fruit and vegetables a day to ensure a healthy vitamin, mineral and fibre intake. Choose fresh or frozen fruit and vegetables in preference to canned, and eat them raw or lightly cooked to preserve nutrients.

Eat frequently

At least 50% of everything you eat should be

Eat sparing

Eat in moderation

Eat frequently

Eat unlimited

carbohydrates. If you view carbohydrates with a degree of suspicion, this might seem high. The high-protein/low-carbohydrate diet (see pages 30 – 31) of the Seventies convinced many of us that potatoes and pasta are fattening. Yet, there are plenty of examples of people who maintain lean physiques on even higher proportions of carbohydrates: in the Far East, for instance, rice traditionally provides around 80% of calories. Obesity has only recently become a problem in Japan, and it is directly related to the introduction of a Western diet that is high in protein and fat, and low in carbohydrates. Medical opinion stands firm: it is easier to store the fat you eat as body fat, than it is to store

carbohydrates as fat. To increase your carbohydrate intake, eat plenty of sugar-free breakfast cereals, bread, pasta and rice (see pages 28 – 29). Wholegrain varieties are preferable as they contain more vitamins, minerals and fibre.

Eat in moderation

Between 10 and 20% of your diet should be protein, which amounts to around two servings a day. The adult daily requirement for protein is probably lower than you think, and most of us eat more than enough protein without even trying. In developed nations, protein deficiency is virtually non-existent. Although children and pregnant women need slightly more, an adult weighing 60kg (132lb) has a daily requirement of only 45g (1½oz). In theory, 200g (7oz) of prawns would provide all the protein needed. In reality, the protein in your diet must come from a wide variety of foods to ensure a balance of essential amino acids (see pages 30 – 31). Protein is present in most foods. Meat and dairy products are high in protein but, as they can also be high in fat, choose lean meat, poultry without the skin, and low-fat cheese and milk. Dried beans, tofu and fish are also good low-fat sources of protein.

Eat sparingly

Fat should make up no more than 30% of your diet. This means foods high in fat should, for the most part, be avoided, as nearly everyone can afford to reduce the amount of fat they eat. But, however desperately you want to lose weight, do not try to cut out fat completely; it is an essential part of a balanced diet. Fat is a component of most foods, so you probably eat much more than you realize. If you are used to a high-fat diet, you may initially miss the flavour, but tastebuds can be educated; cut down gradually on the fat you eat, and you may even find you don't like it any more. Also, keep an eye on the type of fat you are eating; two-thirds of it should be unsaturated (see pages 32 – 33).

How to read food labels

The information on the back of a packet of food is not just there to entertain you during breakfast; it is there to help you make informed decisions about what you eat. Most packaging carries a list of ingredients and a nutritional table. Learning how to make sense of labelling will allow you to see at a glance whether what you are eating is nutritionally sound.

How to get it right

Ingredients Listed according to amount, the ingredient that comes first is there in the largest quantity. Study a few food labels, and you may be surprised at the information they contain: vegetable oil can be high in the list of ingredients for cakes, biscuits and even breakfast cereals. Food manufacturers have been known to use misleading descriptions, so beware: vegetable oil can often mean coconut oil. Not exactly a vegetable and, unlike all other vegetables, it is high in saturated fat.

HOW TO CALCULATE WHAT'S IN FOOD

With some basic mathematics, you can use the nutrition table to work out the percentage of fat and carbohydrates in a packet of food.

■

If the nutritional table shows 50g (1.8oz) wholemeal bread has: 1g (0.04oz) fat, 22g (0.8oz) carbohydrates and 114 calories.

$\frac{1}{50}$ x 100 = 2% of the bread is fat
$\frac{22}{50}$ x 100 = 44% of the bread is carbohydrates.

The nutritional table

This describes the nutritional quality of the product you are buying. It doesn't have to list all the ingredients, just those that are relevant to calorie intake, and they can be listed per serving or per 100g.

Calories Shown as either "kcalories", "kilojoules", or "energy", the figure given tells you how many calories there are, but doesn't indicate where they come from. Food can be low-calorie, yet still be mainly made up of refined sugar and fat.

Protein Shown only as a total amount, you have to look at the list of ingredients to see for yourself if the protein comes from animal or vegetable sources. Protein is present to some degree in almost all food.

Carbohydrates These are sometimes sub-divided into sugars and starches, or "refined" and "complex" carbohydrates. Alternatively, sugars can be listed under the general heading of "carbohydrates", which makes it difficult to check the amount of refined sugar added. Sugar provides energy but is of little nutritional value.

Total fat content This is often followed by a figure showing how much of the total amount of fat is saturated. All fat is equally fattening but unsaturated fat is a healthier choice. Beware: reduced-fat foods sometimes can contain up to 40% fat.

Additional information Some nutrition tables list elements that are known to have implications for health, such as sodium (a component of salt), vitamins and minerals, or fibre. The presence of fibre probably indicates that the carbohydrates are unrefined, although this isn't always the case.

Using common sense

When there is no nutritional table, you have to use your own judgement to estimate the likely fat content. Remember the following:

Fat makes food greasy If your fingers are greasy after handling food, you can assume that it is high in fat. Sugary foods tends to make your fingers feel sticky.

Saturated fat tends to solidify At room temperature, saturated fats harden, which can be quite useful: when stews and soups are left to cool, the fat forms a crust over the top that can be easily removed, substantially lowering the fat content.

Fatty foods "melt down" Animal fats melt when heated. The fat in sausages and hamburgers, for instance, melts when they are cooked and can be drained away or dabbed with kitchen towel.

Cut down on processed foods Pies, cakes, biscuits and ready-meals are often laden with hidden sugars and fats.

Seven Point Plan

Now that you know the facts about dieting, you can understand why weight loss does not – cannot – happen overnight. Losing weight is about eating sensibly in the long term, not about starving yourself. You need a strategy that you can stick to: a well-formulated plan rooted in fact and not in fiction.

1 Modify your diet by striking the right balance between the types of food you eat (see pages 38 – 39). This means cutting down on fat and increasing the amount of carbohydrates in your diet. The Good Food Guides (see pages 42 – 49) will help you to do this.

2 Eat little and often. Convention dictates we eat three square meals a day, with a break of several hours between. We aren't designed to go so long without food, which is why the snack-food industry prospers. Rather than three big meals, eat three smaller meals, and two high-carbohydrate, low-fat snacks.

3 Don't skip meals. It encourages your body to crave food and, if it becomes something of a "forbidden fruit", the desire to eat can be overwhelming, regardless of how hungry you really are. Eating sufficient carbohydrates, in small, frequent meals, will reassure the body it will be fed regularly.

4 Cut down on alcohol. Sorry about this, but alcohol does contain a lot of calories which are very rarely put to good use. Although it may initially appear to perk you up, alcohol has a sedative effect and will make you much less inclined to use the energy those calories provide.

5 Drink more water. It does not make you fat, and few people drink enough. Neither tea or coffee are particularly good for quenching thirst, as they both contain caffeine, which is a diuretic and speeds up the rate of urine loss. Substitute bottled water, or try fruit or herbal teas. If you're not used to them, try several before you decide you don't like them; fruit flavours are less bitter than herbal teas.

6 The Total Fitness Plan (see pages 50 – 91) will help you get rid of excess body fat. Do it at least three, and preferably five, times a week. The strength training section (see pages 64 – 79) can, on occasion, be omitted, but never miss out the aerobic section.

7 Persevere. Don't be tempted to fall for any of those dieting fantasies: starving yourself as punishment for overindulgence won't help. We all go off the rails sometimes, so don't hate yourself for it. One chocolate doesn't make or break a diet but eating the whole box because you didn't have one when you wanted it probably will. Getting it nearly right each day is better than perfection once a week.

The Good Food Guides

The Good Food Guides are designed to steer you safely through the day by offering nutritious suggestions for breakfast, lunch, dinner and snacks. They are full of ideas for spicing up a high-carbohydrate, low-fat diet, but you don't have to follow them slavishly.

This is not a cookery book – there are no specific recipes for controlling your weight and there are plenty of other books available that can tell you how to prepare delicious, low-fat meals. Neither is it a diet book, at least not in the traditional sense: it doesn't dictate a detailed weekly menu and then leave you to guess what to do when you reach the end of it. A diet will not work if it's repetitious and boring, or if you are forced to eat foods you do not particularly like. If it is going to be successful, an eating plan has to prepare you to make your own informed decisions about what to eat in the long term.

As long as you stay within the guidelines, you can adapt the suggestions that follow to suit your taste. Once you are armed with the information you need to balance your diet, it is easy to make the right choices.

The Good Breakfast Guide

Probably the most important meal of the day, breakfast is – literally – the breaking of the overnight fast. Although you have been sleeping, your body has been using energy to stay alive and carry out repairs. Breakfast is its chance to refuel.

Research reveals two interesting facts about breakfast

1 People who skip breakfast are more likely to be overweight than those who regularly eat breakfast.

2 In tests, people who were given a high-carbohydrate breakfast voluntarily chose to eat less later in the day.

It is especially important to start the day with a high-carbohydrate meal. It will give you the energy you need to get to work, and will enhance your mental ability when you get there: research has shown that children who eat a high-carbohydrate breakfast do better in school tests than those who have a high-fat breakfast, like bacon and eggs. Try some of the following ideas:

- Unsweetened muesli with low-fat yoghurt and fruit
- Any high-fibre cereal without added sugar
- Dried fruit – apricots, figs, dates and prunes
- Low-fat yoghurt or fromage frais with puréed apple, flavoured with cinnamon or nutmeg
- Porridge with blackberries or other soft fruit
- Wholemeal toast or low-fat bagels with a low-sugar/high-fruit jam – gradually cut out butter, or try to find a low-fat, unhydrogenated spread
- Fruit juice – a good source of vitamin C, carbohydrates and fluid
- English muffins with grilled pineapple or mango
- Banana, melon, and orange juice blended with yoghurt
- Grilled tomatoes on toasted soda bread
- Pancakes with sliced banana and low-fat yoghurt
- Limit yourself to a single cup of tea or coffee with reduced-fat milk, or try herbal or fruit teas.

The Good Lunch Guide

Lunch is a meal we often eat on the run. Very few of us have the time to sit down for a three-course feast. This isn't necessarily a bad thing: digesting large meals often makes you feel lethargic. It makes more sense to have a lighter lunch and a reasonably sized snack (see pages 48 – 49) either side of it.

Plan ahead

If you know you are going to be away from home during the day, without access to good, healthy food, it is worth preparing your lunch in advance; fill a Thermos with soup, make a salad or sandwich, and take it with you.

Sandwiches

There are so many types of bread available now, such as ciabatta, focaccia, pitta, naan, rye and soda bread, that the sandwich is no longer a boring option. Choose wholemeal bread over refined, white bread, as the fibre makes you more full. Opt for sandwiches and rolls with more bread than filling. Fillings should be low in fat, so avoid ordinary mayonnaise, butter, margarine, fatty meat or cheese. Good fillings include:

- Grilled chicken or turkey, watercress and cucumber
- Low-fat cream cheese or fromage frais with mint and sliced fresh apricots
- Low-fat hummus, grated carrot and chopped fresh coriander leaves
- Mashed banana with cottage cheese
- Low-fat mozzarella, sliced tomato and fresh basil
- Low-fat vegetable pâté.

Jacket potatoes

Easy to cook, jacket potatoes provide plenty of long-term energy. They are high in fibre and contain only a trace of fat. Baked sweet potatoes are a good alternative. Fillings should be low in fat, so avoid butter and cheese, and choose from the following:

- Tuna, sweetcorn, red kidney beans, celery, spring onion and low-fat mayonnaise

■ Baked beans spiced with Tabasco, Worcestershire sauce or chilli sauce, and chopped tomato
■ Grilled tomatoes, fresh herbs and seasoning
■ Cottage cheese with a spoonful of pesto
■ Lightly sautéed mushrooms in garlic with chopped chives and a spoonful of plain yoghurt
■ Salsa: chopped pineapple, peppers, chilli, fresh herbs and lemon juice.

Pasta
Naturally low in fat and high in carbohydrates, pasta is an excellent source of energy, but choose your sauce carefully; pasta is easily transformed into a high-fat dish by adding a cheese- or cream-based sauce. Try the following options:
■ A tomato-based sauce, with finely sliced courgettes or other raw vegetables, tossed with pasta, a small spoonful of olive oil and freshly ground black pepper
■ Pesto sauce: although it contains quite a lot of oil you need to use so little that it is not a bad choice
■ Steamed broccoli and chopped fresh chilli sautéed in a little olive oil.

Rice
Substantial and filling, rice can make a complete meal in itself when it is combined with a few other ingredients. Couscous or bulghar wheat are equally good, but brown rice has more fibre, vitamins and minerals than white rice. Try some of the following recipe ideas:
■ Add raisins and a few almonds to saffron rice
■ Stir blanched spinach leaves and diced, grilled chicken into rice that has been cooked in a stock made with garlic, cumin seeds and turmeric
■ Tuna, chopped fresh chillies and tomatoes and fresh basil stirred into cooked rice.

Soup
Serve with bread that is preferably wholemeal. Try the following combinations:
■ Cook sliced onion in a little oil, add a selection of vegetables – carrots, celery, courgettes, peppers, peas, tomatoes, potatoes – add vegetable stock, season, and cook until all the vegetables are tender. Blend to make a creamy, filling soup
■ Add canned beans – chick peas, cannellini beans, lentils – as a nutritious supplement to the above
■ Add sliced spring onions and fresh ginger to vegetable stock, pour over cooked egg noodles and sprinkle with coriander. Tofu adds a low-fat source of protein to this soup.

Salad
Although salads are a good source of vitamins and cancer-preventing nutrients, you should avoid adding fatty meat, fried croutons and avocado, which (for a fruit) is surprisingly high in fat. Similarly, salads are easily turned from a nutritious lunch into a source of fat by adding spoonfuls of dressing. The following are low-fat combinations:
■ High-carbohydrate foods like corn, kidney beans, lentils, chick peas, rice or pasta, added to chopped peppers, mushrooms, onion, celery and fresh herbs
■ Watercress or fennel mixed with sliced oranges
■ Toasted sunflower seeds or sesame seeds sprinkled over a mixed leaf salad, dressed with balsamic vinegar or lemon juice
■ Grated carrots, combined with grated fresh ginger, chives, lime juice and a few drops of sesame oil.

Soup is delicious and makes a nutritious and substantial lunch. Serve it with plenty of wholemeal bread.

The Good Dinner Guide

If you are cooking for yourself, it is easy to ensure that the food you eat is low in fat and high in carbohydrates. When you eat out, stick to the same criteria – avoid foods that are obviously fatty, like cream- or cheese-based sauces, or anything fried.

Meal planning

Base meals around carbohydrate foods, like pasta, rice and potatoes, rather than adopt the traditional approach, with meat as the central feature. Serve the following dishes with plenty of vegetables, grilled, steamed or roasted, or a large mixed salad:

Pasta Serve pasta with tomato or vegetable sauces, instead of high-fat meat or cream sauces. For a simple fresh tomato sauce, lightly brush halved tomatoes with a little olive oil and roast in the oven for 30 minutes. In a food processor, blend the roasted tomatoes with chopped chilli, garlic and basil leaves, and stir into cooked pasta.

Rice Brown rice is the most nutritious of all the varieties of rice and is packed wiith vitamins, minerals and fibre. You can cook brown rice in a vegetable stock with sliced dried apricots. Then fry sliced onion in a little olive oil, and add ground cumin, coriander and chilli powder. Roast cubes of pumpkin or sweet potato that have been lightly brushed with oil, and mix with the rice and spices.

Fish Fillets or steaks of fish can be given an oriental flavour: blend together fresh ginger, soy sauce, lemon juice, spring onion and five-spice powder in a food processor until they form a thick paste. Spread over the fish and grill.

Meat Choose lean cuts of meat and trim off any obvious fat before cooking. Use a cooking method that allows the fat to drain away – grilling or roasting, rather than frying. Dab meat with kitchen towels to soak up any excess fat after cooking. Marinades add flavour to meat without adding a lot of extra fat. For a Moroccan-inspired marinade, combine lemon juice with chilli powder, cumin, paprika and a splash of olive oil. Marinate cubed lean lamb, chicken, or fish for at least one hour before grilling.

Poultry

Choose grilled chicken or turkey. Much of the fat in poultry lies under and in the skin, so remove it before cooking to prevent the fat seeping into the flesh as it cooks. The marinades for meat or fish are equally good with poultry.

Pizza

This can make a well-balanced meal, especially when the crust is thick or deep-pan; it is the pizza topping that can be a problem. Avoid meat, keep high-fat cheese to a minimum, and choose vegetable-based toppings instead. Top a pizza base with a fresh tomato sauce or a thin layer of pesto sauce or olive paste, and add thinly sliced mushrooms, peppers, tomatoes and garlic. Sprinkle with fresh or dried oregano or fresh basil. Drizzle with olive oil, if desired, and bake in the oven until crisp and golden.

Vegetables

Most of us do not eat enough vegetables, yet they contain vital vitamins and minerals, and they are very low in fat. Allow vegetables to form the central part of a meal: stuff peppers or aubergines with a mix of onions, peppers, courgettes, herbs and tomatoes cooked in a little olive oil. Bake in the oven for one hour and serve with rice. For variety, add tuna, sweetcorn, chick peas or black-eye beans. Puréed vegetables also make simple and nutritious sauces and soups.

Potatoes

To replace chips, cut potatoes into wedge shapes, lay on a baking tray, season, and drizzle with a little olive oil. Bake in the oven for one hour, until golden. Alternatively, thinly slice potatoes and combine with sliced onion, tomato, fresh rosemary and garlic in a baking dish. Pour over some vegetable stock, cover with foil, and bake in the oven for one hour.

Room for dessert

If you eat a main course that is high in carbohydrates, you will probably find that you do not have room for dessert. However, if you are still hungry, here are some healthy options:
■ Fresh fruit – melon, kiwi fruit, grapes
■ Low-fat yoghurt mixed with fruit and sunflower seeds, or sweetened with a little honey
■ Baked apple stuffed with raisins, dates or dried apricots and a little honey
■ Low-fat rice pudding, sprinkled with grated nutmeg
■ Puréed mango or pineapple mixed into plain yoghurt or low-fat fromage frais
■ Fruit purée - for a simple fruit sauce, blend frozen raspberries and strawberries in a liquidizer (add a little caster sugar if the fruit is very tart). Pass the purée through a sieve to remove the seeds, and serve warm or cold with low-fat yoghurt or fruit sorbet
■ Stewed dried fruit – figs, dates, apricots, apples, sultanas, peaches and pears
■ Meringues with fruit and low-fat fromage frais.

Be imaginative in your use of vegetables – they can form the central part of a meal.

The Good Snack Guide

The point of "snacking" is to bridge the gap between main meals and keep blood sugar levels constant. When your blood sugar fluctuates, so does your energy. To avoid this, you should snack on foods where the calories come from complex carbohydrates, not from fat.

Healthy snacks

Many snack foods are very high in fat. We all underestimate how much we eat, and it is easy to overlook the odd handful of peanuts now and then, but that odd handful can add considerably to the total amount of fat you eat. To avoid temptation, create a "safe" environment in your home or work-place by surrounding yourself with plenty of low-fat foods to snack on. If you feel an irresistible craving for something indulgent, it's probably better to go for a sweet treat rather than a fatty one.

Fruit The perfect snack food, fruit even comes ready-wrapped. Where fruit is concerned, there are no restrictions; no fruit (except avocado) is more fattening than any other. Fruit contains practically no fat at all. It is mainly carbohydrates, at least 50% water, and is also high in vitamins.

Dried fruit A compact source of sweetness as well as vitamins and minerals, dried fruit also provides valuable fibre. Dried apricots, raisins, prunes and sultanas are high in iron and potassium.

Raw vegetables Often overlooked as a snack food, this is probably because most vegetables need some preparation before they are eaten. In fact, once they are washed, many vegetables can be eaten raw. They are a good source of carbohydrates, and contain plenty of vitamins, minerals and fibre.

Pitta bread Low-fat hummus, salad, or grilled vegetables mixed with a little pesto sauce or olive tapenade, make delicious fillings for pitta bread.

Rice cakes Nibble them plain, or top with absolutely anything – vegetables, fresh fruit, jam or cottage cheese.

English muffins and scones These are a healthy source of carbohydrates, but are often turned into a high-fat snack by adding butter and cream.

Muffins and scones have a natural sweetness, so try them on their own, or top them with soft fruit, such as strawberries, raspberries or blueberries, and a spoonful of low-fat Greek yoghurt.

Sandwiches and rolls make an excellent high-carbohydrate snack.

If you really crave butter, try to switch to a low-fat spread. These contain about half the fat of butter, but choose one that is unhydrogenated (see page 33), as it is much better for your health.

Bagels Versatile and convenient, bagels can be bought in either sweet or savoury varieties. Onion or pumpernickel bagels can be eaten with a thin layer of low-fat cream cheese, cottage cheese with chives or spring onion, or low-fat vegetable pâté. Sweet bagels, like cinnamon and raisin, do not need much in the way of topping and are perfect toasted with sliced banana or low-sugar, high-fruit jam.

Pretzels An excellent source of carbohydrates, but avoid those that are heavily coated in salt.

Popcorn A healthy snack, as long as the popcorn is not coated with oil, butter or salt. Try making popcorn yourself and flavouring it with paprika, soy sauce, Tabasco or, for a sweet alternative, cinnamon or nutmeg. Avoid the ready-made, caramel-coated variety: the coating is pure refined sugar.

Low-fat biscuits Usually lower in fat than normal biscuits, but check the label as many low-fat biscuits are loaded with refined sugar to compensate for the lack of taste. The calories are often just as high – they just come from a different source. Choose biscuits that are as close to crackers as possible.

Sandwiches An excellent high-carbohydrate snack, as long as the filling is low in fat. For filling ideas, see pages 44 – 45.

Breadsticks These can be eaten on their own, or dipped into low-fat hummus or tzatziki.

Yoghurt All yoghurt is made with milk, but this is often where the similarity ends. It can be made with whole or skimmed milk and sometimes has added sugar, cream or other flavourings. Look at the label, as the fat content of yoghurt can vary from 0.2g (0.01oz) per 100g (3.6oz) in low-fat yoghurt to 9g (0.3oz) per 100g (3.6oz) in full-fat Greek yoghurt. Plain yoghurt can be flavoured with fresh or dried fruit, fruit purée, nutmeg, cinnamon, or used as a low-fat salad dressing. Low-fat fromage frais and crème fraîche are now also widely available.

49

Total Fitness Plan

I am no stranger to exercise – I have been
dancing for most of my life – but the first time
I decided to exercise for *fitness*, I felt as if I was
gatecrashing a private party.

Fitness has become a bit exclusive: you probably think you
have to buy the right gear, join a gym, or hire a personal
trainer if you're serious about getting fit.

In fact you don't need to do any of these things. All you
need to get fit is a good pair of trainers, the right advice,
and a healthy dose of determination. It will all feel a little
strange at first, but bear in mind an old Norwegian
saying: "The mile across the doorstep is the longest".

Getting the Right Gear

There are no hard and fast rules about what to wear when you exercise, unless you intend to take up competitive athletics. In some ways, the most important thing is to feel comfortable. However, as all physical exercise involves sweating – you're going to get wet – some clothes are more suitable than others.

Keeping warm, staying cool

The evaporation of sweat is the body's cooling mechanism. In windy weather, when evaporation is rapid, you risk cooling down too much. The trick is to wear "breathable" clothing that allows sweat to evaporate yet keeps you warm throughout your work out (see side bar). Always wear socks: the Achilles' tendon is never very warm, and a cold tendon is at risk of injury. There is also a practical concern – without socks, sweat quickly rots shoes.

WARM WEATHER

Shorts or track pants and a loose T-shirt.

This is the only weather when shorts are suitable: sweating limbs are best covered up. In intense sunshine, use a sweat-resistant sunscreen to avoid getting burnt.

■

COOL WEATHER

Track-pants and a top of moisture-transporting fabric, such as polypropylene.

You can add a sweatshirt, and (if it's windy) a breathable windbreaker.

■

COLD WEATHER

Moisture-transporting fabric on the legs and upper body.

You can cover this with track-pants and a thin wool layer, like an old sweater. You may need a breathable windbreaker, gloves, and even a woollen hat.

Trainers

To avoid the risk of injury, you should always wear good shoes: this may be the one expense necessary before you can begin. Appropriate shoes are especially important if you plan on jogging.

Bike

For general training, choose a "hybrid" bike. Mountain bikes are really for serious off-road cycling, although "slick" tyres will make them smoother for road use.

Helmet

Never cycle without a helmet and visible clothing. Both are essential.

A firm footing

If you're not used to physical activity, exercise will put an unfamiliar strain on your joints, muscles and tendons. It is vital that you give them as much support as possible by wearing the best trainers that you can afford; don't be tempted to go out in your old school plimsolls (hang on to them though, they provide some valuable information).

Go to a specialist shop and ask for a shoe designed to support your particular type of feet. Take your old shoes with you – they will provide clues as to the sort of trainers you should buy as a replacement.

There are basically three types of feet (see right): flat, "pronating" feet that roll inward, high-arched "supinating" feet that roll outward, and "neutral" feet that are more or less straight. When the feet roll either way, the shoes have to compensate. Pronating feet need "straight-lasted" trainers with good arch- and medial support. Supinating feet need trainers with good arch- and lateral support, and with especially

good shock absorbency, as these feet can be rather rigid. All trainers should be snug, but not tight, and should have good shock absorbency. Unless you intend to run only on dry pavements, avoid smooth-soled shoes, which will be slippery in wet or muddy conditions. Try several pairs before you decide – don't just go for the ones with the best colour scheme. Trainers should be chosen with the feet, not the eyes.

Pronating feet will wear trainers out along here

Supinating feet will wear trainers out along here

WIND CHILL

However warm the temperature, wind speed can have a dramatic effect on how warm you feel. This is known as the "wind-chill" factor. Cyclists should pay particular attention to wind chill, as cycling into the wind increases its cooling effect.

Chin-up bar

Fix a bar just beyond your maximum reach, so it can be used for the hanging stretch. Always check it is secure before use.

Elastic band

There are several types available – choose an inexpensive, basic version made of good-quality rubber.

Bike stand

If you already own a bicycle, this is a cheaper option than buying a purpose-built stationary exercise bike.

Heart-rate monitor

This provides an easy way of checking that you exercise at the right intensity. Choose a basic, inexpensive model.

When To Exercise

It doesn't matter what time of the day you exercise. Although some experts claim that a morning work out raises the metabolic rate and keeps it elevated for the rest of the day, others have found no evidence of any "after burning" effect. Ultimately, it comes down to practicalities. You have to find a space in the day that suits you.

Eating and exercise

Fitting exercise around meal times requires a little planning. You obviously don't want to work out feeling hungry, nor do you want to feel bloated. When you eat is almost as important as what you eat. If you are exercising primarily to burn fat, it is especially important that you do not eat just beforehand. In response to food, the pancreas releases the hormone insulin, which temporarily prevents fat being used as a source of energy.

A question of timing

Digesting a large meal takes several hours, and during this time you won't feel very energetic. There are two reasons for this: firstly, blood is diverted to the stomach to digest the food, so there is less blood available to carry oxygen to the muscles. Secondly, the pancreas releases insulin, and this may make you feel lethargic. The brain requires a constant level of sugar in the blood, and insulin helps to regulate this. When food is digested, the sugar it contains is absorbed into the bloodstream, and the blood-sugar level increases. To counter this, insulin is released to "push" this sugar into the muscles and liver. The consequent drop in blood sugar may bring about a temporary feeling of tiredness. Refined sugar, which releases its energy in one great surge, causes the insulin to overcompensate, which can lead to bouts of dizziness.

You should allow at least two hours between eating and exercise so that you aren't affected by any dips in energy levels. If you've eaten sufficient carbohydrates, you'll have plenty of stored energy available. Work outs lasting less than 90 minutes rely entirely on stored fuel; it's only when you exercise for longer than this that food eaten immediately before or during exercise starts to provide energy.

If you choose to work out first thing in the morning, it can be difficult to fit in breakfast beforehand. Have some fruit or a glass of fruit juice 30 minutes before you start; this will be enough to get you going. Be sure to eat breakfast afterwards.

Energy drinks

Marketing men are a little unscrupulous when they use the word "energy", failing to mention that "low calorie" means low energy, or that "energy" drinks provide energy because they are high in calories.

If you are ill, energy drinks can be very useful, and if you're running a marathon, they can be a lifeline. But if your main objective is to burn fat, energy drinks may not be a good idea, as the sugar content causes the pancreas to produce insulin. While the insulin level in the blood is high, fat cannot be used for energy. If you feel listless or lethargic, take a look at your diet and your lifestyle. Don't imagine you can open a bottle and instantly solve the problem.

The Pre-exercise Plan

Unless you're very fit, it's not a good idea to launch into exercise without a little preparation. Most importantly, leaping directly from the sofa to a 30-minute work out puts you at risk of injury. Even if you escape this, you will ache so much from the unfamiliar activity that you would probably give up on day two.

The three starting levels

Depending on your general fitness, your body takes at least two weeks to adjust to any increase in activity. During this time, the overriding concern is injury prevention. Don't worry that you're not burning fat: it is more important to strengthen your muscles, tendons and ligaments so that you can eventually follow the Total Fitness Plan without interruption from injury. Be sure to complete Level 3 before you move on to the fitness plan.

Where to begin

Every novice exerciser starts from a different level – be honest with yourself, and choose the one that best describes your general fitness. Finish each fitness session with a light stretch (see pages 58 – 59). When you have completed one level, move on to the next. Once you have completed all three, you are ready to start the Total Fitness Plan.

It's also a good idea to start increasing your general level of activity during the day. This will give a much needed boost to your metabolism. Any of the following can be easily incorporated into your daily routine:

■ Cycle or walk to work.
■ If it is not possible to walk all the way, park further from the office, and walk the last couple of miles.
■ Get off the bus or tube a few stops early. You might also save money!
■ Walk up stairs instead of taking the lift or the escalator.
■ Don't use the car for short trips – walk them instead.

LEVEL 1 YEARS OF NEGLECT	*Unable to walk up a flight of stairs without stopping. Two weeks of the following:*
	■ *45 seconds of slow walking* ■ *15 seconds of fast walking* *Alternate between these for 5 minutes daily. Add 1 minute every second day. Finish each session with the light stretch.*

LEVEL 2 UNFIT	*Out of breath after climbing a flight of stairs. Two weeks of the following:*
	■ *1 minute of slow walking* ■ *1 minute of fast walking* *Alternate between these for 10 minutes daily. Add 1 minute every second day. Finish each session with the light stretch.*

LEVEL 3 FAIRLY FIT	*No restrictions in day-to-day activity. Two weeks of the following:*
	■ *1 minute of slow walking* ■ *30 seconds of easy jogging* *Alternate between these for 10 minutes daily. Add 1 minute every second day. Finish each session with the light stretch.*

The Fitness Plan

TOTAL FITNESS PLAN

It consists of six
parts: the "six pack"
of fitness:

■

WARM UP

■

LIGHT STRETCH

■

THE AEROBIC ELEMENT

■

COOL DOWN

■

STRENGTH TRAINING

■

FULL STRETCH

Easy to follow, safe and effective, the Total Fitness Plan is designed to allow you to make your own decisions about the type of exercise you want to do and where you'd like to do it. The only real expense is the cost of a good pair of shoes, although if you want to join a gym, there is nothing to stop you: running on a treadmill is just as effective as running outdoors, except the scenery isn't quite as good.

A well-equipped gym offers the option of machines for strength training but I have become quite adept at finding very effective substitutes: body weight provides tailor-made resistance, and working against it is an excellent way to build strength. You will need an elastic exercise band, but these are not expensive, and you can even use an old bicycle inner tube. A sturdy tree branch can double as a chin-up bar, and a park bench is useful for stretching, as well as for chair dips, abdominal and hamstring exercises.

The Total Fitness Plan works equally well for weight loss and weight maintenance. You need to do it at least three, and preferably five, times a week. The more you do it, the more fat you will burn, but don't forget that the body needs an occasional day off. It is a fitness package to last a lifetime and contains everything you need to lose body fat, maintain and build muscle strength, improve posture and benefit health.

Warm Up

Don't be tempted to skimp on your warm up. It's an essential part of your work out. Until you're properly warm, your muscles and tendons are much less pliable, and therefore less able to cope with the demands of exercise. Exercising without a good warm up significantly increases your risk of injury.

Increasing the temperature

Most materials are more flexible when they are warm: elements as diverse as metal and wax can be moulded once their temperature is increased, and human tissue is no different. You often see people trying to "stretch" before they start their work out but, until the connective tissue in the muscles is warm, stretching is much less effective.

Increasing the pace

Warming up is not only about the muscles in your arms and legs: the heart is also a muscle. A good warm up should raise the heart rate gradually to the level when it can pump enough oxygenated blood around the body to meet increasing demand from the working muscles. Until then, exercise has to be anaerobic (without oxygen) and the build up of lactic acid will make your legs feel tired (see page 20). Don't let this put you off: the muscles will very soon be supplied with oxygen and lactic acid will be recycled. Remember, the beginning is always the hardest bit.

The most efficient way to warm up is also the simplest: start the activity you intend to do at a very gentle level, and increase the pace over about 5 to 10 minutes. For example, if you are going to run, begin by walking for a few minutes, then step up the pace until it becomes a fast walk/easy jog. You can also alternate between two minutes of walking and two minutes of jogging. If you are cycling, start in the easiest gear, and shift up one or two gears every minute. Some types of aerobic exercise may not adapt so easily to become a warm up, but you can safely substitute the walking/jogging formula instead.

Warming up gently introduces the muscles to the movements they are about to do. In addition, co-ordination improves after a few minutes of practice, thereby reducing the risk of injury.

A warm up that uses "large" muscle groups, like the thighs and hamstrings, will obviously be more effective, as it works the heart harder: large muscles need more oxygen than smaller ones. An effective warm up should bring on a light sweat, and leave you breathing hard, but not gasping for breath. If you are warm already, exercise will be effective from the outset.

Light Stretch

Now that you're warm, you should gently stretch before going on to your aerobic exercise. Stretching gradually increases muscle length and flexibility, and long, flexible muscles are less prone to injury. Stretching also acts as a "check point": use it to test that everything is working smoothly before you continue with the next section.

LIGHT STRETCH

See pages 80 – 91 for detailed information on the stretches. For now, they need only be done once on each side:

- INNER THIGH
- HIP FLEXOR
- FRONT THIGH
- HAMSTRINGS
- UPPER CALF

Gently does it

You don't need to push too hard at this point – the full stretch will come later. Choose a suitable spot, with something like a bench to hold on to, and don't pause for too long between the stretches. The light stretches should take no more than a couple of minutes – you don't want to lose the effect of your warm up.

The stretches

All the stretches in the Total Fitness Plan have been chosen because they predominantly stretch muscles that span two joints. They focus mostly on the muscles that attach to the pelvis and spine, as good mobility in this area is important in preventing lower-back pain.

Without muscles, we would be completely immobile. Joints are only made to move by shortening the muscles that cross them. Any repetitive action (the definition of exercise) involves contracting the muscles over and over again, which can make them become

tight. Stretching after exercise counteracts this, gently elongating the muscles while they are still warm. When the two-joint muscles are tight and shortened, they can pull unevenly on the joints and lead to problems.

Stretching also serves as an opportunity to check that all the different parts of your body are in working order. Any increase in the amount of activity you do will inevitably leave the muscles feeling a little stiff and tired the next day; it is the recovery from stiffness that makes the muscles stronger. If you have any twinges above and beyond this, you should not continue to exercise.

In case of injury

Any fitness plan should put safety first, so you should not be at any risk. Accidents do, however, happen and over-enthusiasm – attempting to run before you can walk – may also put a strain on muscles, tendons and ligaments that aren't used to exercise. If you are unfortunate enough to injure yourself don't try to "run it off". If you catch an injury straight away, it will take less time to heal. Stop immediately and remember one word, ICE:

Ice, if available, should be applied immediately and firmly to the injury. Use a wet cloth between the ice and bare skin to prevent ice "burn".

Compression will prevent swelling if it is done immediately. Tie a scarf, T-shirt, or anything else you can lay your hands on, firmly around the injury.

Elevate the injury above the level of the heart to further reduce the swelling that may occur. Discontinue exercise and seek medical advice as soon as possible.

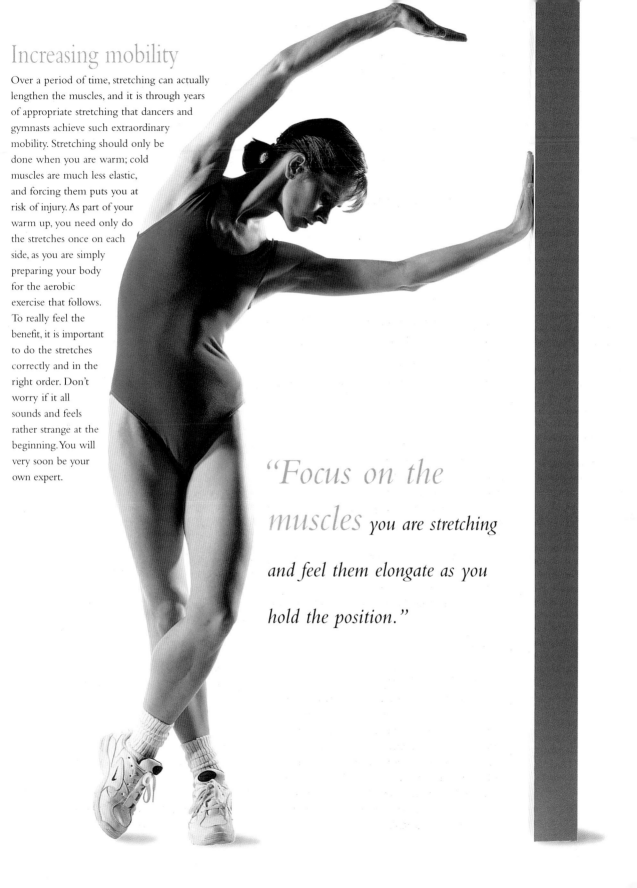

Increasing mobility

Over a period of time, stretching can actually lengthen the muscles, and it is through years of appropriate stretching that dancers and gymnasts achieve such extraordinary mobility. Stretching should only be done when you are warm; cold muscles are much less elastic, and forcing them puts you at risk of injury. As part of your warm up, you need only do the stretches once on each side, as you are simply preparing your body for the aerobic exercise that follows. To really feel the benefit, it is important to do the stretches correctly and in the right order. Don't worry if it all sounds and feels rather strange at the beginning. You will very soon be your own expert.

"Focus on the muscles you are stretching and feel them elongate as you hold the position."

Aerobic Exercise

The aerobic element is the part of your work out designed to burn fat. To achieve this effectively, you have to keep it up for at least 20 minutes, at 60 – 70% of your heart's maximum capacity. Only then, when exercise is of the right intensity and duration, will the energy you use come from body fat.

Starting out

When you begin, you may find that brisk walking is enough to raise the heart rate to 60 – 70% of its capacity, especially if you are not used to exercise. As you get fitter, your heart, like the rest of your muscles, will become stronger, and you will need to increase the pace to push your heart rate to the right level.

Staying in the target zone

As exercise has to be of the right intensity to burn fat, it is important to work out your personal target zone before you start (see pages 22 – 23), and to keep within it. At first, you need to take your pulse at regular intervals to check that your heart is working at the right level. After a while, you will begin to recognize this level, using pace and breathing as indicators, and you won't need to test it quite so often. If you want to be really sure that you are within your target zone, you can buy a heart rate monitor (see page 53).

A defining characteristic of aerobic exercise is that it can be sustained for long periods of time. If you can't keep going, it's probably because you've pushed your heart rate too high. Slow down to a walking pace, and gradually speed up again when it has returned to the target level. Whatever you do, to burn a signficant amount of fat, you must keep going for at least 20 minutes.

If at first you find it difficult to train at a consistent pace for 20 – 30 minutes, try interval training (see tint box, below). Alternating between walking and jogging is the easiest form of interval training and you can use the same formula for any type of activity. This type of training is often more enjoyable, and can also be gentler on the joints than keeping a steady pace.

INTERVAL TRAINING

- *Once you have warmed up, jog until your heart rate reaches 70% of your maximum capacity (see pages 22 – 23).*
- *Slow down the pace to a walk until the heart rate drops to 60% of its maximum.*
- *Step up the pace until the heart rate reaches 70% again.*
- *Continue to alternate between the two for the duration of your work out.*

Choosing your exercise

There are several types of aerobic exercise, and you can choose whichever you like. Your heart doesn't know what type of exercise you are doing; it will only register the fact that your muscles require more oxygen. The "ideal" exercise for burning fat is the one that suits you best, although varying the activity from time to time will reduce the risk of over-using specific joints.

Brisk walking Probably the perfect exercise when you first start out, especially if you're very overweight. It's safe, familiar, low in impact and easy to keep up.

Cross-country skiing If you have access to snow, this is an excellent form of exercise. Cross-country skiers are regularly shown to have the highest fitness levels of all athletes, and relatively low levels of body fat. Cross-country skiing uses all the major muscle groups in the arms and legs, and is very low in impact. Many gyms have exercise machines that simulate cross-country skiing.

Cycling A good alternative to jogging. When cycling, the body weight is supported, so it's gentler on the joints. It does require some equipment – a helmet and visible clothing – but lots of people already own a bike. You do need to be mindful of the wind-chill factor. In bad weather, you can cycle indoors with the aid of a bike stand, which converts your bicycle into a stationary exercise bike (see page 53). These are quite inexpensive and can be bought at a good cycling shop.

Exercise your imagination

Depending on the type you choose, aerobic exercise may or may not be all-weather. It is perfectly possible to run or cycle when it's raining, but if you don't like the idea of getting wet, you can (with a little imagination) adapt most aerobic exercise to be done indoors.

If it's possible, try to find a way to incorporate aerobic exercise into your existing daily routine. This isn't as hard as it sounds and there are several ways in which it can be included (see page 55). One in three households, for instance, owns a bicycle, yet only one in three of those bicycles is ever used. If you have one hidden away, get it out and put it to good use. I would imagine that if everyone who lives within striking distance cycled to work instead of using the car, obesity, road congestion and pollution could be cut in half at a stroke.

Jogging This is arguably the ultimate aerobic exercise as it requires no equipment (other than a good pair of shoes) and works many of the large muscle groups. However, it probably isn't appropriate for absolute beginners, and it does increase the impact on the joints.

Mini trampoline Jogging can be done indoors, on the spot, with the help of a mini trampoline. This is very useful when it's raining, and very gentle on the joints. You can do any aerobic work out on a mini trampoline, and they are especially useful if you prefer to exercise to music.

Rowing The obvious downside to rowing is that you need either a boat or a rowing machine to do it. If you have access to either, it's a great form of exercise. As you do it sitting down, it is a non-impact activity, and works the large muscle groups in both the upper and lower body. You need to take it easy at the beginning, as it can be hard on the lower back.

Running in water This is much harder than it sounds – the effort of moving against the water's resistance makes it a very effective work out for the heart. As you are more or less weightless, it's a good choice if you have any problems with your joints.

Swimming A non-weight bearing, non-impact exercise which works all the major muscle groups against the resistance of the water. The only drawback may be that the cool water keeps the body temperature down, making it less effective in burning fat. It also requires access to a pool or suitable open water.

5-minute Cool down

Like the warm up, the cool down is a part of the Total Fitness Plan that you may be tempted to skip. Don't: it is as important as the warm up. Just as you raised your heart rate to the target level before you began, you must now bring it down again.

A proper cool down will lower body temperature and help guard against any aches and pains.

Easing the pace

To cool down, you simply reverse your warm up. Gradually slow down the pace until your heart rate returns to normal. Whichever type of exercise you have been doing, you can use jogging as a cool down: start out at a moderate pace, and slow to a walk over five minutes.

Strength Training

STRENGTH TRAINING
Follow the order in
which the exercises
are listed.

∎

ABDOMINALS
BACK EXTENSIONS

∎

CHAIR DIPS
HAMSTRINGS

∎

BICEPS
ARABESQUE

∎

INNER THIGH
DELTOID

Strength training helps weight control by maintaining and even increasing muscle mass, which keeps the metabolic rate high. It also improves posture and reduces the risk of injury in daily physical tasks. The strength training will not in itself burn fat, which is why it is the only part of the Total Fitness Plan that can, on occasion, be omitted.

The exercises that follow are paired so that you can work one set of muscles while another set recovers, and you should do them in the order in which they appear. Start with the first of each pair given: focus on the muscles you are targeting, and continue to work until they are too tired to do the exercise correctly. Switch to the second exercise of the pair and follow the same procedure. You may want to repeat both the exercises before moving on.

It is more important to do the exercises accurately than to aim for a specific amount of repetitions (completed movements) but a number you can work toward is suggested for each exercise. You should eventually try to repeat each pair three times. The length of time it takes to achieve this will vary enormously from person to person. As a rough guide, it should take about three months to double the number of repetitions you can do. Don't worry if it takes longer: quality is more important than quantity.

Abdominals

The abdominals are a very important muscle group, as strong abdominals support the spine. They also help to keep the stomach flat. Unless the abdominals are exercised with the hips and knees bent and supported, the psoas does most of the work and the lower back is put under strain.

THE ABDOMINAL MUSCLES criss-cross the abdomen, with their main attachments at the lower ribs, breast bone and pelvis.

1 *Lie on your back,* with your calves resting on the seat of a chair, and your knees and hips supported at a 90° angle. Gently cup your hands around the back of your neck.

Do not hook the feet in place

Keep the hips and knees bent at a 90° angle

2 *Contract your stomach muscles* and raise your head and shoulders slightly off the ground.

Do not pull the head forward with the hands

3 *Without touching the floor,* "crunch" up and down by moving your chest toward, then away from your knees. Start with 2 sets of 5, building up to 3 sets of 15. After each set, lower your body down gently and stretch out fully, with your arms above your head for a count of 15.

Feel the muscles contract in the stomach

Maintain the position of the feet and legs

Loosely cup your hands behind your head, as shown above. If you find it more comfortable, cross your arms over your chest instead.

CAUTION

Do not pull the head forward.

Do not hook the feet in place.

Do not twist the spine to target the "oblique" muscles. It can be dangerous, and this exercise works them sufficiently.

Back Extensions

This exercise targets most of the muscles in the back, especially the erector spinae muscles which run prominently down both sides of the spine. Back extensions are important because they balance the strength of the abdominals and improve posture. If either the back or abdominal muscle groups are weak, there is a risk of lower back pain and injury.

THE ERECTOR SPINAE MUSCLES are attached to each vertebra down the spine, from the base of the skull to the pelvis.

1 *Lie face down, flat on the floor, with your arms stretched straight out above your head.*

Lift both arms and legs at a steady rate

2 *First tighten your buttock muscles, then lift your arms and legs steadily, so that your nose and knees are just off the ground. Hold this position for a count of 3, then gently lower your body. Relax for a count of 3, then repeat. Start with 2 sets of 3 lifts, building up to 3 sets of 10 lifts.*

Do not raise the head above the arms

CAUTION

Always tighten the buttocks before commencing Step 2, to protect the lower back.

Do not lift the back or the legs too high off the ground.

The upper body lifts until the nose is just off the ground

"Back extensions

will help to give you a dancer's

strength in your back."

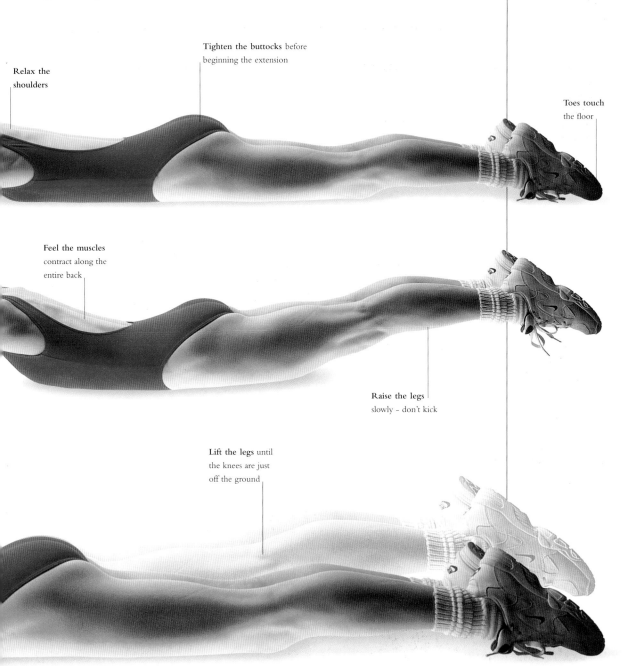

Relax the
shoulders

Tighten the buttocks before
beginning the extension

Toes touch
the floor

Feel the muscles
contract along the
entire back

Raise the legs
slowly – don't kick

Lift the legs until
the knees are just
off the ground

Chair Dips

Chair dips offer an excellent alternative to the more usual push-ups as they work a wider combination of muscles. This is a very safe way of exercising the latissimus dorsi in the back, as well as the triceps and pectorals, because it provides some traction for the spine. Chair dips will improve muscle tone in the torso, and help firm the back of the upper arms.

THE TRICEPS MUSCLE is situated along the back of the upper arm, and crosses both the shoulder-joint and the elbow.

1 *Support yourself* with both hands on the seat of a chair, so that your arms are slightly behind you. Suspend your weight on both arms and stretch your legs out in front of you.

Do not lock the arms

Your body should just clear the seat

Keep the legs straight

Rest on the heels

CAUTION

Do not lower yourself too far at first, or you might strain the shoulder joint.

2

Bend your elbows and gently lower your body as far as feels comfortable. Push back up in one smooth movement, until your arms are straight again. Start with 2 sets of 3 repetitions, building up to 3 sets of 15.

Feel the muscles working in the back of the arms

Feel the muscles working on both sides of the back

Keep the body vertical

Do not lower yourself too far until the exercise is more familiar

Hamstrings

Strong and flexible hamstrings contribute to good posture, and work together with the abdominals to protect the lower back. Since most aerobic exercise, such as running and cycling, strengthens the quadriceps at the front of the thigh, it is important to balance this with selective training of the hamstrings.

THE HAMSTRINGS is the collective name for the group of muscles in the back of the thigh. They originate at the back of the pelvis and attach below the knee.

Double hamstring

1 *Lie flat on the floor* with your arms at your sides for support. Place both heels of your feet on the seat of a chair, with your knees bent at right-angles.

2 *Lift your pelvis* high off the floor by pushing your weight down onto your heels. Hold the position briefly.

Feet rest on the heels

Spread the arms slightly for stability

Knees and hips are bent at a 90° angle

3 *Move your pelvis* up and down, without letting your bottom touch the ground. Rest and repeat. Start with 2 sets of 3 repetitions, building up to 3 sets of 7.

Keep the arms flat on the ground

Do not let the bottom touch the floor

CAUTION

This is quite a tough exercise. Do not attempt too many repetitions until accustomed to it.

One-legged hamstring

*You can progress to this exercise once you are able to
complete the double hamstring with ease. Lie as before, but
with your right heel on the seat of the chair and your left
leg pointing upward. Lift your pelvis high off the floor by
pushing down through your right heel, and move up and
down as before, without letting your body touch the ground.
Lower yourself down and repeat with your other leg. Start
with 2 sets of 6 repetitions, building up to 3 sets of 14.*

Keep the
leg vertical

Push the weight down
through the heels

Keep the arms flat
on the ground

Biceps

This exercise can be performed in any one of three ways. The chin-up works the biceps and the brachialis muscles, while the inclined chin-up and the arm-curl, with its elastic resistance, offer an easier alternative which women may find easier to execute. For the chin-up, you will need a bar or a tree branch, and for the arm-curl you will need an elastic exercise band (see page 52).

THE BICEPS and THE BRACHIALIS MUSCLES oppose the TRICEPS. Together, they provide bulk and strength in the upper arm.

Chin-up

Let the body weight fall evenly on both arms

Grip the bar with your hands shoulder-width apart and your palms facing backward (see right).

Relax the legs

Lock the thumbs around the bar

Keep the body straight

Underhand grip

Use an underhand grip, with the palms facing toward you, not an overhand grip.

1

2 *Pull your body up* as far as you can and hold the position momentarily. Slowly lower yourself and repeat. Start with 2 sets of 2 repetitions, building up to 3 sets of 7 repetitions.

CAUTION

If the chin-up feels too hard, do arm-curls until you have increased your strength.

Inclined chin-up

1 **Fix the bar** at waist height. Grasp it with an underhand grip (see left), hands shoulder-width apart, keeping your body straight and your heels on the ground.

Check that the body is in line

Keep the body straight

Heels are hip-width apart

2 **Pull yourself up** as high as possible and hold momentarily before slowly lowering yourself. Start with 2 sets of 2 repetitions, building up to 3 sets of 7 repetitions.

Arm-curl

1 **Place your right foot** slightly in front of your left and fix the elastic beneath it. Hold the elastic in your right hand, with your elbow bent and the elastic tight enough to give slight resistance.

Hold the back straight

Ensure that the elbow remains close to the body

Keep the legs apart for stability

Elastic exercise band

Adjust elastic tension so that the repetitions are just possible

2 **Bend your elbow** and pull the elastic up to your shoulder. Hold the position briefly, before slowly lowering your arm. Start with 2 sets of 6 repetitions on each arm, building up to 3 sets of 10 repetitions.

CAUTION

Do not let the elastic slip from beneath the foot.

Arabesque

This is one of the most common positions in ballet. Here, it is borrowed from the dance class and adapted for use in strength training. Ballet technique is not always appropriate for non-dancers, but the combination of turn-out and lift in the arabesque is particularly effective in working the gluteal muscles and firming the buttocks.

THE GLUTEAL MUSCLES make up the bulk of the buttocks. They connect the pelvis and the femur bone in the thigh.

1 *Stand with your feet together, facing the back of a chair with both hands resting on it for support.*

2 *Turn out your left foot as far as it will go and check that your hips are still facing forward. With your left hand, feel the muscles in your buttock working.*

3 *Keep your left foot turned out and lift the leg behind you as high as it will go without tilting your pelvis.*

4 *Gently raise and lower your leg until the muscles are tired, then repeat the movement with your other leg. Start with 2 sets of 6 repetitions, building up to 3 sets of 15 repetitions.*

CAUTION

Do not lift the foot too high, or you may strain the lower back.

"Ballet dancers spend half their working lives in arabesque, so this exercise comes as second nature to me."

Do not arch the back

Movement comes from the hip

Feel the muscles contracting in the buttock

Keep the foot turned out

Inner Thigh

The adductors are the muscles on the inside of the thighs that bring the legs together – you feel them work when you cross one leg over the other. This exercise has a strong aesthetic factor, as it helps to firm the inner thighs. It also develops the specific strength needed in sports such as football, skiing and rollerblading.

THE ADDUCTOR MUSCLES stretch between the knee and the pelvis, on the inside of the thigh.

Keep the pelvis facing forward

The foot remains flexed throughout

Use the hand for support

1 *Lie on your side,* and support your head on one hand. Cross your left leg over your right knee, so that your foot is positioned flat on the floor.

Do not twist the torso

"Feel the muscles

working by resting your hand on

your leg from time to time."

Do not allow the
body to twist as
the leg moves

**Keep this
leg** straight

2

Lift your lower leg as high as possible and gently
move it up and down without letting it touch the
ground. Start with 2 sets of 6 repetitions on each
leg, building up to 3 sets of 20.

Feel the muscle work
along the inner thigh

Deltoid

A large, triangular muscle, the deltoid covers the shoulder and is used to lift the arm. By lifting the arm sideways, against elastic resistance, you work as much of the muscle as possible in one movement. This exercise tones the shoulders, strengthens the arms, and improves the look of the upper body. You will need an elastic exercise band (see pages 52 – 53).

THE DELTOID MUSCLE originates from the collar bone and shoulder blade and attaches to the humerus, the bone of the upper arm.

The arms should start level with the hips

Elastic under slight tension

Bend the knee slightly

Stand in a lunge position, so that your right leg is slightly bent and a step in front of your left leg. Lock the elastic under your right foot. Lift your arms to the side, until the band is taut.

The palm faces away from the body

Raise the arms slightly in front of the body, not directly to the side

Do not arch the back

Raise your arms up and outward until they form a wide "V" shape above your head. Hold briefly, lower and repeat. Start with 2 sets of 6 repetitions, building up to 3 sets of 10 repetitions.

CAUTION

Check that the elastic does not slip.

Keep the __wrists__ straight

__The arms are lifted__ slightly to the front of the body

Hold the __body__ straight

__The elastic__ should not be so tight that you cannot complete the repetitions

"This is a wonderful way

of toning the shoulders."

Stretches

THE STRETCHES

Do each stretch on
both sides of the body,
then repeat.

■

INNER THIGH

■

HIP FLEXOR

■

FRONT THIGH

■

HAMSTRING

■

UPPER AND LOWER
CALF

■

SIDE

■

CAT/HANGING
(WHOLE BODY)

Never underestimate the value of stretching: it increases muscle length and flexibility and long, supple muscles are less prone to injury. Short muscles, however strong they are, will always be a source of problems, as they cannot cope with such a wide range of movement. Stretching after your work out is especially effective, as aerobic exercise raises your body temperature, and the connective tissue of muscles is much more elastic when it is warm.

When practised correctly, stretching should be a pleasant and not a painful experience. Take the stretch position gently, breathe in, and then sink deeper into it as you breathe out. Focus on the muscle you are stretching and feel it relax as you hold the position for a count of 10. Do the exercises in the order in which they are listed, and be sure to stretch both sides of the body equally. You should repeat the stretches as instructed.

Do not bounce: it stimulates a protective mechanism in the muscle that causes it to tighten as a defence against injury. Your flexibility will increase over a matter of weeks, not overnight, so never try to force your body; stretching is one of those things you just can't rush.

Inner Thigh

The adductors, a group of muscles on the inside of the thigh, are used to bring the legs together. A healthy back depends on a good range of movement in the hip joint, and if the adductors are tight, they can limit mobility.

THE ADDUCTORS stretch between the knee and the pelvis, and are located on the inside of the thigh.

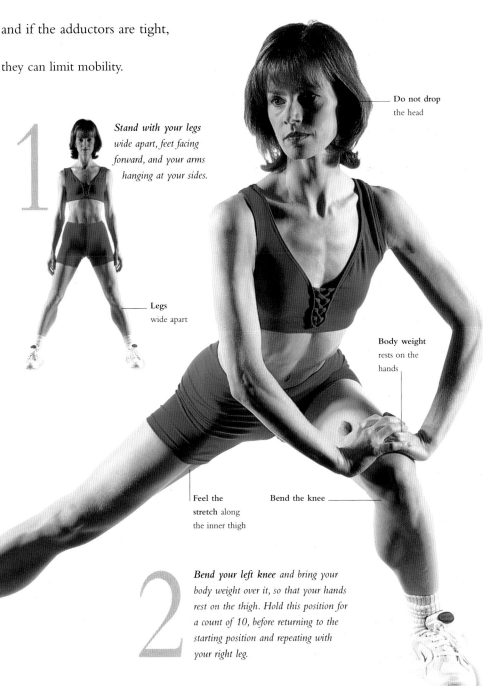

1 *Stand with your legs wide apart, feet facing forward, and your arms hanging at your sides.*

Legs wide apart

Do not drop the head

Body weight rests on the hands

Feel the stretch along the inner thigh

Bend the knee

2 *Bend your left knee and bring your body weight over it, so that your hands rest on the thigh. Hold this position for a count of 10, before returning to the starting position and repeating with your right leg.*

CAUTION

Do not lean forward. Push against the thigh to ensure that you do not round the back.

81

Hip Flexor

The psoas muscle, commonly called the hip flexor, lifts the leg in front of the body – an action used, for instance, in running and walking. Due to its complex relationship with the hip and spine, it rarely gets to stretch out fully. A tight psoas pulls on the lower spine, contributing to back pain. Combining a flexible psoas with strong abdominal muscles protects the lower back.

THE PSOAS MUSCLE (the "p" is silent) runs between the femur, or thigh bone, and the lower spine.

1 *Kneel on your right knee with your hands resting on your front thigh.*

Straight spine

2 *Extend the position by pushing your pelvis toward the ground. Feel the stretch in your right psoas as you push against your front thigh.*

Keep the back straight

Ensure the lower leg is vertical

Push the pelvis downward

Cushion the knee with a folded towel if necessary

CAUTION

To protect the spine, push the pelvis as far as possible toward the ground before beginning step 3.

Stretch the arm
to form an arc

3

Balance yourself *with your left hand, and raise your right arm up and backward to complete the stretch. Hold for a count of 10, then return to the starting position and repeat on the other side.*

Arch the spine
gently backward

"Fine tune all of these

stretches to maximize their

effectiveness for your

own physique."

Feel the stretch
deep in the thigh

Front Thigh

The rectus femoris is one of the four quadriceps muscles in the front of the thigh. Of the four, it is the only muscle that crosses the hip and knee joints. Any action that involves lifting a straight leg in front of you – kicking a ball for instance – will activate the rectus femoris. If it is tight, it may tilt the pelvis forward, causing problems in the lower back.

THE RECTUS FEMORIS MUSCLE is located along the front thigh and stretches from the knee to the hip.

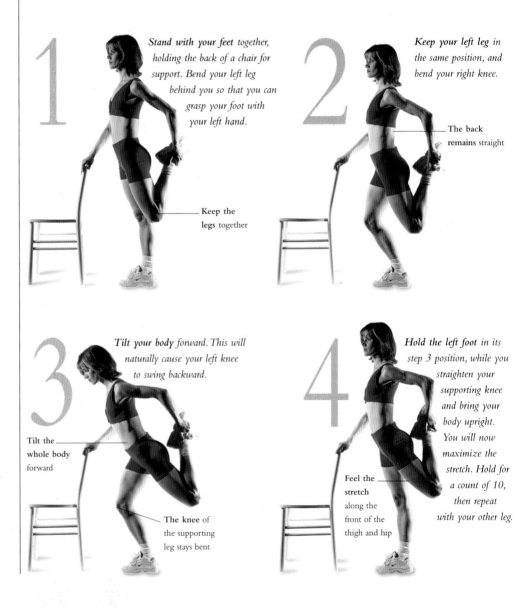

1 *Stand with your feet together, holding the back of a chair for support. Bend your left leg behind you so that you can grasp your foot with your left hand.*

Keep the legs together

2 *Keep your left leg in the same position, and bend your right knee.*

The back remains straight

3 *Tilt your body forward. This will naturally cause your left knee to swing backward.*

Tilt the whole body forward

The knee of the supporting leg stays bent

4 *Hold the left foot in its step 3 position, while you straighten your supporting knee and bring your body upright. You will now maximize the stretch. Hold for a count of 10, then repeat with your other leg.*

Feel the stretch along the front of the thigh and hip

Hamstrings

The group of muscles in the back of the thigh is collectively known as the hamstrings. They are used to bend the knee and lift the leg behind the body. Tight hamstrings are easily injured, and can also be an indirect cause of back pain.

THE HAMSTRINGS originate at the back of the pelvis and attach below the knee.

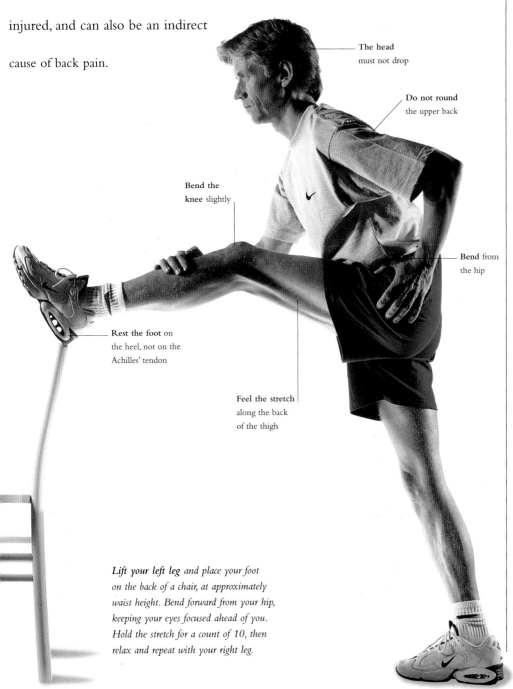

The head must not drop

Do not round the upper back

Bend the knee slightly

Bend from the hip

Rest the foot on the heel, not on the Achilles' tendon

Feel the stretch along the back of the thigh

Lift your left leg and place your foot on the back of a chair, at approximately waist height. Bend forward from your hip, keeping your eyes focused ahead of you. Hold the stretch for a count of 10, then relax and repeat with your right leg.

CAUTION

To avoid stressing the sciatic nerve, keep the raised foot relaxed, the knee slightly bent, and look straight ahead.

85

Upper Calf

The calf has two major muscles: the gastrocnemius and the soleus. The gastrocnemius is the rounded, upper part that provides the powerful push-off used in walking, running and jumping. If tight, it can lead to problems with the Achilles' tendon, to which it is connected, and can distort the alignment of the foot.

THE GASTROCNEMIUS MUSCLE is in the upper part of the calf. It originates at the femur and inserts at the heel.

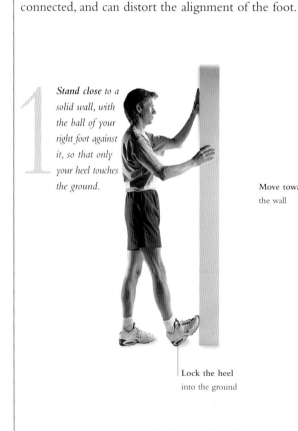

1 *Stand close to a solid wall, with the ball of your right foot against it, so that only your heel touches the ground.*

Lock the heel into the ground

2 *Keeping your front knee straight, push forward, so your hips move toward the wall, and the heel of your hind foot lifts slightly off the floor. Hold for a count of 10, then repeat on your left leg.*

Move toward the wall

Ensure the knee is straight

CAUTION

Move gently from step 1 to step 2, as this technique can generate considerable force.

Lower Calf

The soleus is the broad, flat muscle in the lower part of the calf. Unlike all the other stretches, which involve muscles crossing two joints, the soleus is a one-joint muscle, and only crosses the ankle. One-joint muscles do not usually cause problems, but the soleus needs special attention because it works so closely with the gastrocnemius.

THE SOLEUS MUSCLE originates in the bones of the lower leg, and combines with the gastrocnemius to form the Achilles' tendon.

Keep the back straight

Lock the heel into the ground

Bend the knee toward the wall

Stretch is felt along here

1 *Stand at arm's length from a solid wall. Place the ball of your right foot against it, so that only your heel touches the ground.*

2 *Stretch the lower calf by bending your right knee and pushing it toward the wall. Hold for a count of 10, then repeat with your left leg Follow this stretch by repeating the upper calf stretch opposite.*

Side Stretch

This stretch elongates the entire side of the body, from the knee through to the fingertips. Its primary function is to stretch the muscles on the outside of the hip, but this is an all-purpose exercise that also targets the muscles that bend the body to the side and the muscles that lie between the ribs.

THE TENSOR FASCIAE LATAE and the OBLIQUE ABDOMINAL MUSCLES lie at the side of the body. The INTERCOSTAL MUSCLES lie between the ribs.

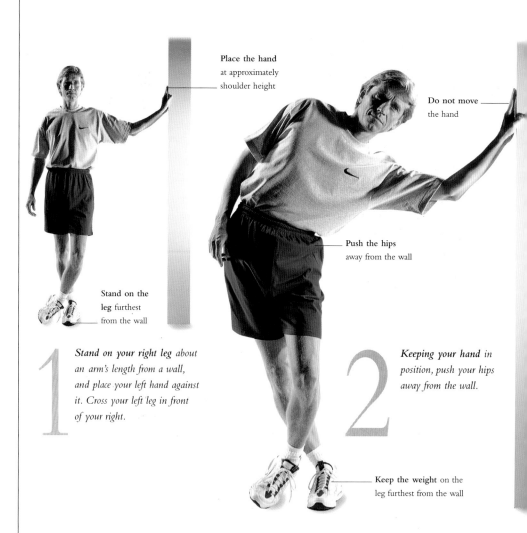

Place the hand at approximately shoulder height

Do not move the hand

Push the hips away from the wall

Stand on the leg furthest from the wall

1 *Stand on your right leg about an arm's length from a wall, and place your left hand against it. Cross your left leg in front of your right.*

2 *Keeping your hand in position, push your hips away from the wall.*

Keep the weight on the leg furthest from the wall

The **palm** of the
hand faces upward

Feel the stretch
along the outside
of the hip and the
side of the body

Do not twist the
body – keep the
hips facing forward

Complete the curve by bringing
your right arm over your head. You
should feel the stretch along the whole
of the right side of your body. Hold
for a count of 10, relax, and repeat
on the other side.

3

Keep the weight on
the supporting leg

Cat Stretch

The spine is made up of 24 individual vertebrae held together by muscles, ligaments and discs. A healthy spine relies on mobility between the vertebrae. When this is limited, back problems can arise. The cat stretch is an excellent way to maintain and even increase mobility in the spine, and so guard against back problems.

THE VERTEBRAE run all the way down the the back, from the skull to the tail bone.

Look straight ahead

Arch the back

Keep both the arms straight

1 *Position yourself on all fours, with your arms in line with your shoulders, and your knees in line with your hips. Look straight ahead, and arch the back downward as much as you can. Once you have reached this position, move on to step 2.*

Relax the head and allow it to drop

Feel the stretch along the spine

2 *Drop your head and curve your spine up as fully as possible, so that your back forms an arc. Try to feel each segment of your spine move. Reach the position, then go back to step 1. Alternate between both steps 4 – 8 times.*

CAUTION

To avoid neck injury, keep looking straight ahead in step 1.

Hanging Stretch

Ever since man decided to walk upright, the spine has been subject to the negative effects of gravity. The hanging stretch helps to counteract this by providing traction for the spine as well as the shoulder joints. If you do not have a suitable bar (see pages 52 – 53), use a sturdy branch on a tree instead.

THE SPINAL COLUMN is made up of the vertebrae and encloses the spinal cord, which it protects.

Lock the thumbs around the bar

Check that the body weight falls evenly on both arms

Hang with your arms about shoulder-width apart. Use an overhand grip, with the palms of your hands facing forward (see right). Hold the position for a count of up to 15.

Relax the legs

Overhand grip

An overhand grip allows you to relax your shoulders. Only the muscles flexing your fingers should be working.

Post-exercise

After you have finished exercising, drink a glass or two of water to replace the fluid you have lost. Eat a high-carbohydrate snack, such as a piece of fruit, to restore your energy. *Do not replace the fat you have just lost!*

Glossary

Aerobic Exercise: Low- to moderate-intensity, long-duration exercise, when energy is supplied using oxygen. Aerobic endurance exercise is the only time when fat can be broken down and used directly as the main source of energy.

Amino Acids: Organic compounds necessary in the formation of protein. Essential amino acids cannot be manufactured by the body and must be obtained from food.

Anaerobic Exercise: High-intensity, short-duration exercise that is fuelled by carbohydrates and does not utilize oxygen.

Blood-sugar Level: The concentration of glucose in the blood.

Body Fat: Storage fat that accumulates under the skin.

Calorie: The unit used to indicate the energy value of foods. This energy is used to fuel the body. It is also now measured in joules (1 calorie = 4.19 joules). A "calorie deficit" is when the body uses more calories than the diet provides.

Carbohydrates: The large group of sugars, starches and dietary fibre that contain carbon, hydrogen and oxygen. Carbohydrates are the main source of energy for all body functions, and are needed to process other nutrients. They are formed by all green plants, which use the sun to turn carbon dioxide and water into simple sugar molecules. They can also be made in the body.

Cholesterol: A substance found in liver, egg yolk and some shellfish. It is also made in the human body, mainly in the liver and kidneys. Cholesterol helps to absorb fatty acids and to make vitamin D and various hormones, including the sex hormones, but surplus amounts of it can be dangerous.

Cramp: Prolonged, painful contraction of the muscles, often caused by the imbalance of salts in the body, but more often as a result of fatigue, poor posture or stress.

Diuretic: Tending to increase the flow of urine from the body.

Endorphins: Hormones produced in the brain that have natural pain-relieving qualities. During exercise their production increases, leading to a general sense of wellbeing.

Energy: Needed for the body to function and be active. Measured in calories or joules, and derived from carbohydrates, protein and fat.

Enzymes: Proteins that accelerate biological reactions.

Fat: A substance made up of fatty acids that is found in both animals and plants. It provides a concentrated form of energy and can be stored as body fat.

Glucose: A simple sugar found in certain foods, such as fruit. All other carbohydrates are converted to glucose before the body can use them as its main source of energy. Glucose can be stored in the liver and muscles, as glycogen, then converted to glucose when needed.

Glycogen: The major carbohydrate that is stored in cells. It is an energy source, made from glucose and is stored chiefly in the liver.

Heart Rate: A measure of cardiac activity, usually expressed as the number of beats per minute (BPM).

Hormone: A chemical substance that is released into the bloodstream and carried to specific receptor sites in the body, where it acts to modify their structure or function.

Insulin: Hormone produced by the pancreas, that regulates the body's absorption of carbohydrates.

Lactic Acid: A vital substance in the production of energy, which is recycled when there is sufficient oxygen available. In anaerobic energy production, it builds up in the cells and limits endurance.

Ligament: A tough band of tissue that connects two bones, or holds organs in place.

Metabolism: The collective term for the chemical changes in living cells, by which energy is provided for vital processes like growth and functioning. The "resting metabolic rate" reflects the energy required to keep the body functioning when it is at rest.

Minerals: A group of inorganic substances that occur naturally in the earth's crust and must be included in the diet. They are important in regulating many bodily functions.

Muscles: Tissues with the ability to contract, causing and allowing movement of the joints.

Obesity: A condition characterized by excessive body fat.

Osteoporosis: A condition in which the density of the bones declines, making them brittle and, therefore, prone to fracture.

Protein: A compound of carbon, hydrogen, oxygen and nitrogen that provides the raw materials (amino acids) for growth and repair. Proteins form the structural material of muscles, tissues and organs. In certain circumstances, protein can be converted into glucose and used for energy.

Repetition: A single, completed movement of an exercise.

Resting Metabolic Rate: See metabolism.

Set: The name for a group of repetitions.

Target Zone: The heart-rate range for a specific exercise intensity.

Tendons: A tough band of connective tissue that connects muscle to another body part, usually bone, and transmits the force that the muscle exerts.

Vertebrae: The bony segments that, together, make up the spinal column.

Vitamins: Organic substances that neither supply energy nor contribute to body mass, yet have a crucial part to play in almost all body processes.

Index

A

abdominal muscles 65, 66, 70, 88
abdominals (strength training) 65
Achilles' tendon 86, 87
adductor muscles 76, 81
aerobic endurance exercise 21, 60–2
    target zones 23, 60
aerobic energy system 21
aerobic exercise 19, 21, 60–2, 92
    adapting for warm up 57
    target zones 23, 60
alcohol 26, 41
amino acids 30–1, 39, 92
anaerobic energy system 20
anaerobic exercise 19, 20, 57, 92
    target zones 23
animal proteins 30
appetite 15, 29
arabesque 74–5
arm-curls 73
arm muscles 68, 72, 78

B

back extensions 66–7
back muscles 66, 68
bagels 33, 43, 49
biceps muscles 72
biceps (strength training) 72–3
bike stands 53, 61
bikes & cycling 52–3
    see also cycling
bingeing 15
biological value 30
biscuits 33, 49
blood sugar levels 14, 29, 54, 92
body fat 92
    body fat/muscle comparisons 12, 13, 14, 16
    energy store & source 16, 18, 21, 26
    fat-burning myths 8, 12, 13
    reduction see permanent weight loss
        & weight control
body wraps 37
brachialis muscles 72
bread 28, 29, 39, 43, 44, 49
breakfast 43

C

caffeine 36, 37, 41
calcium 35
calf muscles 86, 87
calorie content
    body's energy stores 16, 31
    carbohydrates 14, 26, 28
    fat 13, 14, 26
    food labelling information 26, 40
    protein 26, 30
calorie deficit 14, 26, 92
calories, general information 26–7
calorific expenditure 26
    during exercise 14
carbohydrates 28–9, 92
    body's energy stores 16, 31
    calorie content 14, 26, 28
    effect on blood sugar levels 14, 29, 54
    food labelling information 40, 92
    fuel for the brain 12, 16, 28, 30, 31, 54
    fuel for energy systems 9, 20–1, 28
    high-carbohydrate breakfasts 43
    high-carbohydrate diet see high-carbohydrate/low-fat diet
    high-carbohydrate snacks 49, 91
    recommended intake 28, 38–9
cat stretch 90
cereals & grains 28, 31, 34, 39, 43, 45
chair dips 68–9
chin-up bars 53, 56, 72, 73, 91
chin-ups 72–3
cholesterol 32, 33, 92
clothing
    exercise 52
    plastic sweat wear 13, 37
cold-weather clothing 52
complete proteins 30
complex carbohydrates 28, 29, 40
cooking techniques, recommended 34, 38, 46, 47
cool down 63
cool-weather clothing 52
cramp 92
cross-country skiing 61
cycling & bikes 52, 53, 57, 61, 62
    as aerobic exercise 61, 62
    as warm up 57
    and wind chill 53

D

dairy products, nutritional content 30, 32, 33, 34, 35, 39
dehydration 36, 37
deltoid muscles 78
deltoid (strength training) 78–9
desserts 47
dietary fibre 29, 40
diets & dieting
    high-protein/low-carbohydrate 31, 39
    myths 7, 8, 10, 12–3
    recommended see high-carbohydrate/low-fat diet
    yo-yo 7, 8
digestion 13, 27, 54
dinner 46–7
diuretics 36–7, 92
double hamstring (strength training) 70
drinks 36, 37, 41, 54
duration, exercise 19

E

eating pattern, recommended 41
elastic exercise bands 53, 56, 73
endorphins 15, 92
endurance exercise see aerobic endurance exercise
energy 92
    measurement see calories
    storage & use 13, 16, 20–1, 27, 54
        protein conversion into glucose 12, 27, 30, 31
energy drinks 54
English muffins 49
enzymes 13, 92
equipment, exercise 52–3, 56
erector spinae muscles 66
essential amino acids 30, 39, 92
essential fatty acids 32
exercise
    calorific expenditure 14
    effect on appetite 15

exercise *continued*
    effect on metabolic rate 14, 27
    effect on muscles 12, 15, 16
    equipment, clothing & footwear
        52–3, 56
    increasing general activity levels, 55, 62
    intensity & duration 19, 22
    myths 12, 13
    osteoporosis prevention 15, 35
    post-exercise advice 91
    pre-exercise plan 55
    role in weight loss & control 14, 15, 18
    when & when not to exercise 54
    see also individual types of exercise
        by name, e.g. aerobic exercise,
        strength training

F

faeces, water loss in 37
fat-burning myths 8, 12, 13
fat content
    calculating 40
    carbohydrate foods 29
    food labelling information 40
    protein foods 30, 31
fat-soluble vitamins 32, 34
fats 32–3, 92
    in the body *see* body fat
    calorie content 13, 14, 26
    cause of obesity 16, 39
    low-fat diet *see* high-carbohydrate/
        low-fat diet
    recommended intake 32, 39
fatty acids 32, 92
fibre, dietary 29, 40
first aid 58
fish 30, 32, 35, 39, 46
flat feet 53
flour 28, 29
fluid balance 36
food
    as energy source 16, 26
    food groups *see individually by name,*
        e.g. carbohydrates
    food labelling information 26, 40
    water content 36
food combining 13
foot types 53
footwear & trainers 52, 53, 56
front thigh, stretch exercise 84
fructose 28
fruit & vegetables
    in meals and snacks 43–8, 91
    nutritional content 28, 29, 30, 34, 35

    recommended intake 34, 38
    water content 36

G

gastrocnemius muscles 86
glucose 28, 92
    protein conversion into 12, 27, 30, 31
gluteal muscles 74
glycogen 28, 92
grains & cereals 28, 31, 34, 39, 43, 45
great protein myth 31
grips, on chin-up bars 72, 91

H

hamstrings 57, 70, 85
    strength training 70–1
    stretch exercise 85
hanging stretch 91
heart activity during exercise 20, 21, 57
heart rate 22–3, 60, 92
helmets, cycle 52
high-arched feet 53
high-carbohydrate/low-fat diet
    dietary guidelines 38–9
    meal guidelines & suggestions 42–9
    replacements for high-fat foods 33
    role in weight loss & control 9, 14,
        15, 18, 24
    seven point plan 41
    see also individual food groups by
        name, e.g. carbohydrates
high-intensity exercise *see* anaerobic
    exercise
high-protein/low-carbohydrate diet
    31, 39
hip flexor muscles 82
hip flexor (stretch exercise) 82–3
hormones 92
hybrid bikes 52
hydrogenated fats 33

I J K

ICE (ice, compression, elevation) 58
inclined chin-up 73
ingredients lists 40
injuries & injury prevention 55, 57, 58, 59

    inner thighs
        strength training 76–7
        stretch exercise 81
    insensible perspiration 37
    insulin 54, 92
    intensity, exercise 19, 22
    intercostal muscles 88
    interval training 60
    iron 35
    jacket potatoes 44–5
    jogging & running 55, 57, 60, 62, 63
    kcals or kcalories 26, 40
    kjoules or kilojoules 26, 40

L

labels, food labelling information 26, 40
lactic acid 20, 57, 92
lactose 28
latissimus dorsi muscles 68
LDL cholesterol 32
lean tissue 92
ligaments 92
light stretch 58–9
long-duration exercise *see* aerobic
    endurance exercise; aerobic exercise
low-fat diet *see* high-carbohydrate/
    low-fat diet
low-intensity exercise *see* aerobic endurance
    exercise; aerobic exercise
lower calf (stretch exercise) 87
lunch 44–5
lung capacity 21

M

marinades 47
maximum heart rate 23
meals
    guidelines & suggestions 42–9
    recommended eating pattern 41
    timing before exercise 54
meat
    nutritional content 30, 31, 32, 33,
        34, 35, 39
    recommended cooking methods 46–7
metabolism & metabolic rate 13, 14, 27, 92
minerals 26, 29, 34, 35, 92
mini trampolines 62
"miracle diets", myths 7, 8, 10, 13
moderate-intensity exercise *see* aerobic
    exercise

monitors, heart-rate 23, 53
monounsaturated fats 32
mountain bikes 52
muscles 16, 92
    body fat/muscle comparisons 12, 13,
       14, 16
    cool down 63
    effect of exercise 12, 15, 16
    effect of stretching 58–9
    energy use 13, 16
    muscle loss 12, 13, 27, 31
    strength training 64–79
    stretches 58–9, 80–91
    warming up 57, 59
    see also individual muscle groups by name,
    * e.g.* abdominal muscles
myths
    dieting & weight loss 7, 8, 10,
       12–3
    great protein myth 31, 92

neutral feet 53
nutritional tables 26, 40
obesity & overweight 7, 16, 39, 92
oils 32, 33
omega-3 fatty acids 32
one-legged hamstring (strength training) 71
osteoporosis 15, 35, 92
overhand grip, hanging stretch 91
oxygen use during exercise 20–1, 57

pasta 28, 29, 31, 39, 45, 46
pectoral muscles 68
permanent weight loss & weight control
    diet/exercise combination 9, 14, 16, 18
    health & other benefits 15
    practical methods 14
    recommended diet *see* high-carbohydrate/
       low-fat diet
perspiration
    insensible 37
    see also sweating
pitta bread 49
pizza 47
plant protein 30–1
plastic sweat wear 13, 37
polyunsaturated fats 22–3
popcorn 49

post-exercise advice 91
potatoes 28, 31, 39, 44–5, 47
poultry 30, 31, 39, 47
pre-exercise plan 55
pretzels 49
pronating feet 53
protein 30–1, 92
    breakdown products 37
    calorie content 26, 30
    conversion into glucose 12, 27, 30, 31
    food labelling information 40
    great protein myth 31, 92
    high-protein/low-carbohydrate diet
       31, 39
    in muscles 16
    recommended intake 30, 39
psoas muscles 82
pulse rate 22–3

quadriceps muscles 70, 84
rectus femoris muscles 84
refined sugars 29, 40, 54
repetitions 64, 92
resting metabolic rate 27, 92
rice 28, 29, 31, 39, 45, 46
rice cakes 49
rowing 62
running & jogging 55, 57, 60, 62, 63

salads 45
salt 35, 40
sandwiches 44, 49
saturated fats 32–3, 40
scones 49
sets 92
shock absorbency, trainers 53
shoes 52, 53, 56
short-duration exercise
    see anaerobic exercise
side stretch 88–9
simple carbohydrates (simple sugars) 28
skiing, cross-country 61
slimming *see* weight loss
snacks 33, 48–9, 91
socks 52
sodium 35, 40
soleus muscles 87
soups 45

soya beans 31
spine & spinal column 66, 90, 91
"spot-reducing" 12, 13
starches 28, 29, 40
starting levels, pre-exercise plan 55
strength training 64
    abdominals 65
    arabesque 74–5
    arm-curls 73
    back extensions 66–7
    biceps 72–3
    chair dips 68–9
    chin-ups 72–3
    deltoid 78–9
    hamstrings 70–1
    inclined chin-up 73
    inner thigh 76–7
stretches 58–9, 80
    cat stretch 90
    front thigh 84
    hamstrings 85
    hanging stretch 91
    hip flexor 82–3
    inner thigh 81
    light stretch 58–9
    lower calf 87
    side stretch 88–9
    upper calf 86
sucrose 28
sugar content
    drinks 36, 54
    food labelling information 40
    reduced-fat foods 33
sugars 28–9, 40
supinating feet 53
sweating 37
    "breathable" clothing 52
    salt loss 35
    sweat pants 13, 37
swimming 62

target zones (target heart rate) 23,
    60, 92
tendons 92
tensor fasciae latae muscles 88
thigh muscles 57, 76, 81, 84
    strength training 76–7
    stretch exercises 81, 84
    see also hamstrings
tofu 30, 35, 39
trainers & footwear 52, 53, 56
trampolining 62
triceps muscles 68, 72

U V W

underhand grip, chin-ups 72
unrefined carbohydrates 28–9
unsaturated fat 32–3, 39, 40
upper calf (stretch exercise) 86
urea 37
urine, water loss in 37
vegetables & fruit
  in meals and snacks 43–8, 91
  nutritional content 28, 29, 30, 34, 35
  recommended intake 34, 38

water content 36
vertebrae 66, 90, 91, 92
vitamins 26, 29, 32, 34–5, 92
walking 55, 57, 60, 61
warm up 57
warm-weather clothing 52
water 36–7
  in muscles 16
  recommended intake 13, 36, 41, 91
  zero calorie content 13, 26
water loss
  during dieting & weight loss 13, 18, 37
  normal 37
water-soluble vitamins 34

weight loss
  myths 8, 12–3
  permanent *see* permanent weight loss
    & weight control
wind-chill factor 53

X Y Z

yo-yo dieting 7, 8
yoghurt 43, 49

Bibliography

Exercise Physiology; Energy, Nutrition and Human Performance, 4th Edition, McArdle, Katch and Katch, Williams & Wilkins, 1996

Manual of Nutrition, 10th Edition, MAFF, 1995

Gray's Anatomy, 37th Edition, Churchill Livingstone, 1993

Töjning av Muskler, I and II, Evjenth and Hamberg, Alfta Rehab Förlag, 1980

Useful addresses

Chin-up bars:

Polar Electro OY, Professorintie 5, 90440 Kempele, Finland.

Polar Electro Inc, 99 Seaview Blvd, Port Washington, NY 11050, USA
Internet: http://www.polar.fi/

Tunturi, Tunturioyörä Oy, SF 20760, Piispanristi, Finland.
Tel: +358 21 603 111   Fax: +358 21 603 323

Cycle stands:

Tacx Cycletrack, Rijksstraatweg 52, 2241 BW Wassenaar, Netherlands.
Tel: +31(0)70 511 9259   Fax: +31(0)70 511 6411

Cycle-Ops Products, 71 West 11th Street, New York, NY 10011, USA.
Tel: +212 924 6724   E-mail: www.cycle-ops.com

Heart-rate monitors:

Polar, Leisure Systems International Ltd.
Tel: +01926 811 611   E-mail: Isisales@Isi.co.uk
Internet: http://www.polar.fi/sampola/

Acknowledgments

Author's Acknowledgements

I should like to record my gratitude to Torje Eike for advice on the text and constant support, and to Dr Paul Pacy for his generous advice. Torje Eike would like to thank Prof. Patrick Salter of Queen Margaret's College, Edinburgh for instilling in him a life-long interest in anatomy and physiology, and David West, MCSP, for his friendship and professional support over the last decade. We would also like to thank Monica Chakraverty and Robert Ford of Dorling Kindersley for unfailing good humour and valuable advice.

Publisher's Acknowledgements

Dorling Kindersley would like to thank:
Sue Bosanko, Lorna Damms, Nicola Graimes, Nasim Mawji, Jill Scott and Sue Sian. Thanks also to John Woodcock for his illustration work. The following food photography is by Clive Streeter: 44, 46, 48.